D1457424

Behaviors in Dementia
Best Practices for Successful Management

Edited by

Mary Kaplan, M.S.W.

and

Stephanie B. Hoffman, Ph.D.

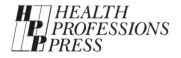

HEALTH
PROFESSIONS
PRESS

Baltimore • London • Winnipeg • Sydney

Health Professions Press, Inc.
Post Office Box 10624
Baltimore, Maryland 21285-0624

Typeset by Barton Matheson Willse & Worthington, Baltimore, Maryland.
Cover design by Four Winds Productions, LLC, Baltimore, Maryland.
Manufactured in the United States of America by
Versa Press, East Peoria, Illinois.

Library of Congress Cataloging-in-Publication Data

Behaviors in dementia : best practices for successful management / edited by Mary
Kaplan, Stephanie B. Hoffman.
    p. cm.
Includes bibliographical references and index.
ISBN 1-878812-43-2
    1. Senile dementia—Treatment. 2. Senile dementia—Patients—Nursing
home care.   I. Kaplan, Mary.   II. Hoffman, Stephanie B.
RC524.B37   1998
616.8′3—dc21   97-44288
                                                                                      CIP

British Library Cataloguing in Publication Data are available from the British Library.

Contents

About the Editors

Mary Kaplan, M.S.W., L.C.S.W., A.C.S.W., is on the faculty of the Department of Gerontology at the University of South Florida, where she teaches courses on mental health and aging and geriatric case management. Ms. Kaplan received her master's degree from the Catholic University of America. She is a licensed clinical social worker and a member of the Academy of Certified Social Workers, National Association of Social Workers.

Ms. Kaplan has worked in the fields of gerontology and health care for more than 20 years as a direct care provider, administrator, and educator. She is a consultant on dementia care, aging programs, and case management services for health care organizations and has conducted workshops on these topics throughout the United States and Canada. As Education Consultant for the Tampa Bay, Florida, chapter of the Alzheimer's Association, Ms. Kaplan provides training in dementia care for program staff in a three-county area.

Ms. Kaplan has published numerous articles and training manuals in the areas of gerontology, health care, and dementia, and is the author of **Clinical Practice with Caregivers of Dementia Patients** and the coeditor of **Special Care Programs for People with Dementia**.

Stephanie B. Hoffman, Ph.D., is Director of Interdisciplinary Team Training and Primary Care Education at the James A. Haley Veterans Hospital in Tampa, Florida. She serves on the Faculty Advisory Council of the University of South Florida Institute on Aging and coordinates regional and national conferences on dementia. She received a master's degree in clinical gerontology and a doctorate in human development and family studies from The Pennsylvania State University.

A life span developmental psychologist, Dr. Hoffman has worked in the field of geriatrics/gerontology for more than 15 years. She has received funded grants to study the communication and management aspects of dementia. At the James A. Haley Veterans Hospital she has trained students and staff in nursing, medicine, psychiatry, psychology, pharmacy, podiatry, social work, speech-language pathology, audiology, occupational therapy, dietetics, physical therapy, and chaplain services.

Dr. Hoffman has conducted workshops on dementia management and team training throughout the United States in continuing education programs and long-term care and other settings. She has published in the areas of geropsychology, dementia, team building, and nonverbal communication, and has coauthored (with C.A. Platt) **Comforting the Confused: Strategies for Managing Dementia** and coedited **Special Care Programs for People with Dementia**

Contributors

Edna L. Ballard, M.S.W., A.C.S.W.
Duke University Medical Center
Box 3600
Busse Building, Room 3510
Durham, North Carolina 27710

Ann Louise Barrick, Ph.D.
Department of Psychology
University of North Carolina-
  Chapel Hill
Chapel Hill, North Carolina 27514

Elizabeth C. Brawley, I.I.D.A., I.F.D.A.
President
Design Concepts Unlimited
PO Box 454
Sausalito, California 94966

Kathleen C. Buckwalter, Ph.D., R.N.,
  F.A.A.N.
Professor, College of Nursing
University of Iowa
101 Nursing Building, 442 NB
Iowa City, Iowa 52242

Linda L. Buettner, Ph.D., C.T.R.S.
Assistant Professor
Decker School of Nursing
PO Box 6000
Binghamton University
Binghamton, New York 13902-6171

Elizabeth J. Brown, R.D.H., M.S.
Edith Nourse Rogers
  Memorial Veterans Hospital
Bedford, Massachusetts 01730

Jiska Cohen-Mansfield, Ph.D.
Research Institute of the Hebrew Home
  of Greater Washington
6111 Montrose Road
Rockville, Maryland 20852

Carly R. Hellen, OTR/L
Director of Alzheimer's Care
The Wealshire
150 Jamestown Lane
Lincolnshire, Illinois 60069

Lisa Kelley, R.N., M.A.
College of Nursing, University of Iowa
101 Nursing Building, 442 NB
Iowa City, Iowa 52242

Peter A. Lichtenberg, Ph.D., A.B.R.P.
Associate Professor of Physical Medicine
  and Rehabilitation
Rehabilitation Institute of Michigan
Wayne State University
  School of Medicine
261 Mack Boulevard, Room 555
Detroit, Michigan 48201

Meridean Maas, Ph.D., R.N., F.A.A.N.
Professor and Chair, Adult and
  Gerontological Nursing
College of Nursing, University of Iowa
101 Nursing Building, 442 NB
Iowa City, Iowa 52242

Susan E. MacNeill, Ph.D.
Assistant Professor of Physical
  Medicine and Rehabilitation
Rehabilitation Institute of Michigan
Wayne State University
  School of Medicine
261 Mack Boulevard, Room 555
Detroit, Michigan 48201

Ellen Mahoney, D.NSc., R.N. C.S.
Associate Professor
Boston College School of Nursing
Chestnut Hill, Massachusetts 02167

Philip D. Sloane, M.D., M.P.H.
University of North Carolina/
  Sheps Center for Health
725 Airport Road, Suite 200
Chapel Hill, North Carolina 27514

Marianne Smith, R.N., M.S.
Geropsychiatric Clinical Nurse Specialist
Abbe, Inc.
3150 E Avenue, NW
Cedar Rapids, Iowa 52405

Patricia A. Tabloski, Ph.D., R.N. C.S.
Associate Professor
University of Connecticut School of
  Nursing
U-26, Room 113
231 Glenbrook
Storrs, Connecticut 06269-2026

Levi Taylor, Ph.D.
Research Institute of the Hebrew Home
  of Greater Washington
6111 Montrose Road
Rockville, Maryland 20852

Rajeev Trehan, M.B.B.S., M.D., M.P.H.
Chief Medical Officer, Knoxville Division
Director of Mental Health
  and Chief of Psychiatry
VA Central Iowa Healthcare System
1515 West Pleasant Street
Knoxville, Iowa 50138

Ladislav Volicer, M.D., Ph.D.
Clinical Director/GRECC
Edith Nourse Rogers
  Memorial Veterans Hospital
200 Springs Road
Bedford, Massachusetts 01730
Professor of Pharmacology
  and Psychiatry
Boston University School of Medicine
Boston, Massachusetts 02118

Karen Williams
University of Connecticut
  School of Nursing
U-26, Room 113
231 Glenbrook
Storrs, Connecticut 06269-2026

Foreword

Behaviors in Dementia: Best Practices for Successful Management is a welcome addition to the professional literature dealing with ways to improve or at least preserve the quality of life of people who are experiencing the steady declines that accompany progressive dementias. The editors and chapter authors are leaders and experts in their respective areas and have much to offer professionals and family members who work with and care for people with dementia. The philosophies, ideas, experiences, and suggestions that they share in this book provide the reader with a good understanding of what we caregivers have learned and how we can be more effective in assisting, managing, and caring for older adults with unique and challenging behaviors. I am equally impressed by the authors' abilities to stimulate ideas and enthusiasm for future applications and interventions. It is a pleasure to be one of the first to read the book because my own professional work has been enhanced by the knowledge that I gained from these authors. Let me explain why.

My professional interests in dementia began in the early 1980s with a primary focus on the multiple burdens experienced by family members caring for loved ones with dementia. Our faculty research team at the University of Utah Gerontology Center joined the growing number of investigators across the United States who wanted to identify the specific stresses, challenges, and needs of caregivers. Since those early days, national attention has shifted toward testing the effectiveness of various interventions. The evolution of our Center's research on caregiving parallels this trend.

Our research clearly identified respite as caregivers' most desired and necessary service. We developed Video Respite, a series of 10 videotapes, to allow caregivers convenient opportunities for brief breaks from the constant demands of people with moderate to advanced dementia. After 4 years of study and an emerging national research program on the effectiveness of Video Respite, the results are very positive for caregivers. Equally important are the less intended but highly promising effects on viewers with dementia—we wanted the videotapes to be engaging and stimulating in order to hold the viewers' attention, but we did not realize just how enjoyable they might be. Although more research is needed to document specific benefits to viewers, it is obvious that the videotapes can make viewers feel better, more cooperative, and less agitated. Several of the chapters in this book helped me to understand more fully why our videotapes were (somewhat unexpectedly) beneficial to viewers. Because of this surprising success we are moving our research in the direction of testing the videotapes' effectiveness as a strategy in behavioral management of people with dementia.

The editors and authors address four elements that I believe are essential for professionals to incorporate in their caregiving, if they have not already done so. The first is multidisciplinary collaboration. The writers obviously recognize and respect that no single discipline can devise effective solutions to the multidimensional, complex challenges of dementia. Second, professionals must understand that many effective interventions and caregiving techniques exist and they should be applied more frequently and broadly. The book also addresses cutting-edge interventions and ideas that deserve wider application. Third, professionals must extend their creative thinking beyond that which already appears to work. Fourth, the most effective interventions are likely to be those guided by theory or conceptual models, which help to make complex situations more understandable. When we develop interventions based on theories we are in a much stronger position to know why particular interventions may or may not work effectively. **Behaviors in Dementia** closely matches my interests in developing and testing more effective interventions for people with dementia, particularly applications that are likely to improve the quality of life of these individuals, their caregivers, and the professionals who work with them. Every chapter in this book contains ideas and suggestions of considerable practical value to me and is likely to have an impact on my work for many years.

Mary Kaplan and Stephanie Hoffman have succeeded in making **Behaviors in Dementia** relevant to me and, I hope, to many others. This book makes sound, practical, and important contributions to the literature on managing challenging behaviors in people with dementia.

Dale Lund, Ph.D.
Director and Professor
University of Utah Gerontology Center

Preface

The growing body of literature on dementia care suggests that much of the behavior exhibited by people with dementia is an attempt to satisfy basic needs and to cope with an often-confusing and frightening environment. The editors have brought together in one volume a compendium of academic knowledge, research, and vast clinical experience that will help professional caregivers understand some of the most common behaviors associated with dementia and that will provide them with effective intervention strategies.

This book supplies interdisciplinary approaches and strategies that have been used successfully to alleviate the problematic behaviors of older adults with dementia. Some of the information contained in this book was presented at the third biennial dementia-specific care unit (DSCU) conference, "Behaviors in Dementia: Strategies for Successful Management." Other leading experts in dementia-related behaviors have added their findings to provide dementia care providers with a wealth of information that addresses a wide range of behavior issues.

The terminology used throughout the book to describe dementia-related behaviors varies. Whereas some authors use the term "problem behaviors," others refer to "challenging behaviors," "disruptive behaviors," "disturbed behaviors," or "difficult behaviors." This inconsistency not only reflects the professional diversity of the contributors but also demonstrates different perspectives on the ways that behaviors in dementia are viewed.

The book begins with a three-chapter look at the foundations, assessment, and care planning methodologies that dictate the types of and approaches to care that are examined in subsequent sections. Then, Section II, "Staff Roles in Caregiving," addresses the roles and responsibilities of staff in preventing and alleviating problematic behaviors, and demonstrates ways in which staff and family members can work together to facilitate managing the behaviors of older adults with dementia. Mary Kaplan discusses the importance of training staff in appropriate methods of behavior management, and Stephanie Hoffman explicates the necessity for staff to use a nurturing approach in caring for their residents/clients and older adults' deep need for it. The role that the mental health consultant plays in prescribing interventions for problem behaviors is critical, and Lichtenberg and MacNeill stress the importance of proper assessment, especially for delerium, and of working well with the interdisciplinary team. The final chapter of this section by Buckwalter and associates examines the relationship between staff and resident/client family members, that they should "partner" to achieve good-quality care for the older adult.

Section III, "Management Strategies," discusses at length the strategies and interventions that are used and are beginning to be implemented to manage the behavior of residents in DSCUs and long-term care settings, although we acknowledge the desire of some professionals, such as Kitty Buckwalter, to shy away from the concept of "managing" behaviors. According to Betsy Brawley in Chapter 8, the environment in which the person with dementia lives is a vital contributor to behaviors he or she may exhibit. She quotes Gene Cohen: "Environmental approaches are not appreciated, even though they often have a faster, safer, and more effective impact than other interventions." Patricia Tabloski and Karen Williams bring clinical and nursing perspectives to their chapter on using music to calm agitated behaviors, and Linda Buettner speaks to the success of activities as an intervention for disturbed behaviors on the DSCU. Ladislav Volicer and his colleagues discuss nonpharmacological approaches to managing behaviors in advanced dementia such as Snoezelen, simulated presence therapy, and others, whereas Rajeev Trehan looks at the latest pharmacological interventions.

Section IV identifies and examines specific challenges that are encountered in the daily care of people with dementia. Carly Hellen addresses the obstacles faced in feeding older adults with dementia by contributing an in-depth table devoted to the cognitive, physical, psychosocial/emotional, and environmental challenges to and possibilities for mealtime success and the interventions that can be used to ensure success. Phil Sloane and Ann Louise Barrick look at bathing and disruptive vocalization and suggest a novel approach to management. In the concluding chapter, Edna Ballard tackles the controversial subject of staff and families' dealing with older adults' sexual behaviors in long-term care, positing that education is the key to effective coping.

We offer our appreciation to the many individuals who cooperated in the process of developing this book. In addition to the chapter authors, we wish to thank our colleagues at the Department of Gerontology, University of South Florida, and the James A. Haley Veterans Hospital. Special thanks goes to Joan Sager for her assistance in reviewing and revising the manuscript.

I

Assessment and Care Planning

1

Care Options

Mary Kaplan, M.S.W., L.C.S.W., A.C.S.W.

The most common behavior disorders affecting older adults are associated with dementia, which causes many of them to lose cognitive and functional abilities. Because individuals with progressive dementia eventually become dependent, they usually require some form of long-term care. Dementia is the most frequent cause of institutional placement of older people in the United States and other Western nations. It is estimated that in excess of 50% of all residents of nursing facilities manifest a dementia syndrome (U.S. Congress, 1992). Some people with dementia also exhibit psychiatric symptoms such as paranoia, depression, delusions, hallucinations, and severe agitation. Before the deinstitutionalization trend in psychiatric care in the 1970s, state mental hospitals were the primary residential care settings housing these individuals. The movement from inpatient psychiatric care to the community mental health model has resulted in fewer care options for people who may have severe behavior problems that require a specially trained staff and knowledge of medication usage in order to manage those behaviors. Often, arranging placement in long-term care settings can be difficult and may not be appropriate if the facility is not prepared to handle psychiatric behaviors.

REGULATIONS AND LAWS GOVERNING LONG-TERM CARE

The implementation of the Omnibus Budget Reconciliation Act (OBRA) Nursing Home Reform Amendments of 1987 and 1990 has changed the framework for

3

serving residents of nursing facilities from an exclusive focus on safety and benef-
icence to a balanced focus that values safety but has added elements of autonomy
and enabled choice. These regulations present a special challenge to service
providers to older adults with behavior disorders related to dementia or mental
illness.

One of the major reforms instituted by OBRA '87 was the development of a
uniform resident assessment system for nursing facilities. The Resident Assessment Instrument (RAI) was implemented in all long-term care facilities participating in Medicare or Medicaid programs beginning in 1990. The RAI consists of
the Minimum Data Set (MDS), the primary screening and assessment tool, and
the Resident Assessment Protocols (RAPS), which specify triggers that identify
potential problems and provide guidelines for the development of care plan goals.
The MDS can be used to identify behavior disorders, document treatment, or
management interventions, and, in some cases, suggest the need for transferring
or discharging the resident to another level of care. The RAPS include several
areas of concern related to behavior disorders: cognitive loss, mood state, psychosocial well-being, behavior problems, psychotropic drug use, and physical
restraints. These areas help health care professionals to make a distinction
between serious behavior disorders and those that can be accommodated more
easily.

Although OBRA '87 provides no special regulations for dementia-specific
care units (DSCUs), some states have made changes in their licensure, certifica-
tion, and survey requirements for DSCUs (Gerdner & Buckwalter, 1996). As of
1996 Iowa, Kansas, Tennessee, Texas, and Washington State added requirements
for DSCUs to their nursing facility regulations. Florida and Rhode Island passed
laws that require all licensed health care facilities that claim to provide special
care to people with dementia to disclose what those special services entail.
Additional states are in the process of developing regulations for DSCUs. The
Alzheimer's Association has published guidelines to provide direction in establishing standards for DSCUs. In 1993 the Joint Commission on Accreditation of
Healthcare Organizations (JCAHO) developed a protocol of standards for DSCUs,
the main thrust of which is that any long-term care facility with a DSCU applying for JCAHO accreditation is required to ensure that their unit is surveyed using
that protocol (JCAHO, 1996).

Laws and standards that regulate other types of residential care settings
are limited and usually do not address the special needs of older adults with
dementia. No federal regulations exist, and state regulations vary for residential
alternatives to nursing facilities such as assisted living, supportive housing, and
residential care homes (Alzheimer's Association, 1994). The lack of regulations
and standards, coupled with the ambiguous distinction between assisted living
facilities and other types of residential care settings, make it difficult to identify
appropriate care options for individuals who are experiencing behavior disorders
associated with a dementing illness.

GUIDELINES FOR CHOOSING CARE OPTIONS

Mrs. Effie Meyer had been taking care of her husband, Jack, age 75, for 5 years in their home. Diagnosed with dementia of the Alzheimer's type, Jack had progressed from being a successful businessman to a confused, disoriented individual who could no longer write his own name. For several years, Effie was able to meet his care needs without assistance, but when care became difficult to manage alone, she enlisted the services of a home health aide to assist with Jack's bathing and to provide some respite so that she could get out of the house for short periods of time. Eventually, Effie found it difficult to manage Jack at home. His behavior became increasingly aggressive. During one incident, he became violent and threw her against a wall. His attention became difficult to redirect, and he began to wander out the door and into the neighborhood whenever Effie took her eyes off him. Medication trials had not been effective, and her home health aide was threatening to resign. At the insistence of Jack's physician and his home health social worker, Effie reluctantly began to investigate area nursing facilities. With the help of the home health social worker, she found a nursing facility dementia care program with a staff who had been trained to manage the behavior disorders that are associated with dementia.

Long-term care includes a range of community-based and institutional services that provide a continuum of care to meet the physical and psychosocial needs of older people. Often, the decision to admit older adults with dementia to a residential setting is made when behavior problems emerge (Hutton, Dippel, Loewenson, Mortimer, & Christians, 1985; Knopman, Kitto, Deinard, & Heiring, 1988; Smallegan, 1985). Behaviors often cited as reasons for placement include the following:

- Agitation, verbal or physical abuse
- Wandering
- Resistance in performing activities of daily living (ADLs), such as bathing or dressing
- Sleep disturbances

The safety and welfare of the individual with dementia and the well-being of the family caregiver should be considered in determining the need for residential placement. Residential care licensure regulations do not guarantee that the special needs of a resident with dementia will be met. Even admission criteria for dementia-specific programs vary and in general are based on the program's philosophy of care, physical environment, and staffing. Many residential facilities are not appropriate for people with dementia who exhibit behaviors such as wandering and agitation because they cannot provide a safe, secure environment and do not have an adequate number of staff who are trained in dementia care. Unfortunately, this information may not be communicated to family members at the time of admission. Often, families are under the impression that placing their relative in a program that claims to provide care for people with dementia means that this care will continue throughout the progression of the disease. Therefore, they are surprised and angry when they are notified that they must make arrangements to remove the resident from the program due to changes in his or her medical, physical, or mental status, or because of his or her disruptive behavior.

Providers of dementia care should have in place admission and discharge policies that include criteria for discharge or transfer and should communicate this information to family members at the time of admission. The following are examples of discharge criteria that can be used in dementia care programs:

1. An unstable or complex medical condition that requires acute or specialized care
2. Functional status that is significantly reduced, resulting in total dependency in ADLs and a high level of care required (e.g., feeding tube, oxygen)
3. A behavior disorder that poses danger to self or others
4. Resident cannot participate in or benefit from program activities because of one of the above situations, misdiagnosis, or improvement in status (Kaplan, 1996)

Many times decisions about care are made in a time of crisis. When a crisis occurs or when a caregiver realizes that he or she can no longer continue to provide care to an individual with a dementing illness, a lack of knowledge about the types of available resources can leave the caregiver uncertain about how to proceed. Table 1 indicates the care options that may be appropriate for individuals who are experiencing challenging behaviors associated with dementia. Table 2 lists the care options that may be appropriate for people with dementia who have a coexisting behavior disorder.

A STRUCTURED DECISION-MAKING PROCESS

Using a structured decision-making process assists health care professionals in helping family members, caregivers, and other individuals to view the situation objectively and make decisions regarding an appropriate plan of care. Step 1 of this process is to include family members who have caregiving responsibilities, as well as those who will be affected by the decision. Step 2 is to involve the person with dementia in the decision-making process, if he or she is capable of participating in the plan of care. Step 3 is to identify any behavior disorders: Have all treatment and management approaches been tried in the present setting? Is the behavior

Table 1. Care options for older adults

Level of care	Early stage	Middle stage	Advanced stage
Home care	Homemaker/companion	Case management services, home health aides	Hospice services
Adult day services	Provides socialization, caregiver respite	Clients must have a caregiver who provides supervision and care when not at adult day center; no medical needs that require skilled care; may help to keep person at home and delay nursing facility placement; look for program designed for people with dementia	
Board and care homes	Assistance with personal care, meals		
Assisted living	Housekeeping services, meals; assistance with personal care and medications; organized social programs, transportation, and recreational activities	Dementia-specific facilities provide increased supervision and therapeutic programs; supervision of medications; look for facilities designed for people with dementia	
Skilled nursing facility	Appropriate only when a coexisting medical condition requires placement	Look for facilities with a dementia-specific program; may not accept people with aggressive behaviors; short-term respite for caregivers	Provides total care; hospice services may be available for people in end stages
Psychiatric hospital, psychogeriatric unit		People with Korsakoff's syndrome, Huntington's disease, or dementia pugilistica whose behaviors are not appropriate for DSCUs	

Table 2. Care options for people with dementia and coexisting behavior disorders

Level of care	Affective/personality disorders	Psychotic disorders	Addictions
Home care	Mental health services	Psychiatric nursing; medication supervision	Inpatient treatment follow-up
Adult day services (early-stage dementia)	Socialization, caregiver respite	Day treatment run by mental health program; must be stabilized by medication	Day treatment; establish social network
Board and care homes (early-stage dementia)	Housekeeping services, meals; assistance with personal care	Aggressive behaviors not accepted; must be stabilized by medication; minimal supervision and activities	Minimal supervision
Assisted living (early-stage dementia)	Housekeeping services, meals; assistance with personal care; supervision of medication	Aggressive behaviors not accepted; supervision of medication; minimal supervision	Minimal supervision; not a treatment facility
Homeless shelter (early-stage dementia)	Temporary placement	Aggressive behaviors not accepted	Temporary placement
Skilled nursing facility (middle-, late-stage dementia)	May be appropriate for people with a medical condition requiring nursing care	Must be stabilized by medication; aggressive behaviors not accepted	No current substance abuse
Psychiatric hospital, psychogeriatric unit		Admission usually restricted to people who are considered a danger to themselves or others	Short-term inpatient treatment may be indicated for acute episodes

really the problem or are there other factors that need to be considered (e.g., family issues)? Step 4 is to consider the following options for care:

- People with dementia may display behavior problems that cannot be managed in a nursing facility setting. Many nursing facilities with DSCUs have admission criteria that deny applicants with severe behavior problems or psychotic disorders. Several types of dementia (e.g., Korsakoff's syndrome, Huntington's disease, dementia pugilistica) are characterized by aggressive behaviors and present challenges in the nursing facility setting. The fact that these residents tend to be younger and physically healthier, combined with possible personality changes and combative behavior, creates a risk of harm to staff and other frail, older residents.
- Most assisted living facilities and board and care homes do not accept people with severe behavior disorders.
- Geropsychiatric units in state psychiatric or veterans' hospitals may accept people with severe behavior problems or psychotic disorders, but beds are limited and, often, residents are admitted on a short-term basis.

Step 5 is to evaluate the following components when choosing a care setting:

- Physical environment
  Exit doors secured
  Fire and emergency policies that reflect the needs of residents with dementia
  Use of camouflage/barriers to discourage entry into restricted areas
  Secured outdoor area
  First-floor location preferred
- Specialized program of therapeutic activities
  Activities provided 7 days a week
  Low-key activities available for residents with sleep disorders
  Use of small groups according to level of cognitive functioning
  Variety of activity choices
  Sensory-stimulation activities and materials
  Emphasis on social interaction and feelings of success
- Flexible nutrition program
  Snacks available 24 hours a day
  Adequate time allowed to eat
  Staff trained to assist with feeding
- Consistent, trained staff with strong administrative support
  Adequate staff-to-resident ratio (recommended: one direct care staff member for every six residents)
  Minimum of 8 hours of training in dementia care
  Evidence of ongoing staff education in dementia care
- Written admission and discharge criteria specific to the dementia care program

- Plan of care that addresses psychosocial and medical needs of people with dementia
    - Continued assessment of changes in residents' medical conditions, functional abilities, and behavior
    - Policies that encourage the involvement of families in the residents' plan of care
    - Use of creative approaches to behavior management, with chemical or physical restraints used only after other methods have proved unsuccessful

Step 6, the final step in the decision-making process, is develop an action plan with assigned responsibilities. An alternative plan should be discussed at this time, with consideration given to the resident's long-term as well as immediate needs. Planning should take into consideration the resident's potential to adjust to a new situation or environment.

ARRANGING CARE AND SERVICES

Once it has been determined what level of care is appropriate for the older adult with dementia, the process of locating and arranging care and services begins. Because of the fragmented U.S. health care and social services systems, it is often difficult to identify what resources are available in the community. Often, behavior disorders relegate individuals to categories that make them ineligible for medical care and/or mental health services. Agencies that provide mental health services may exclude someone with dementia, whereas health care facilities often deny admission to a person with a psychiatric illness.

Choosing the appropriate level of care for a person with dementia is made more difficult by the fact that many individuals have several coexisting disorders. Just as a person may have more than one type of dementia, they may also have a dual diagnosis such as "dementia/depression." Dividing the increasing numbers of older people with behavior disorders into diagnostic categories has been useful in making recommendations for treatment or management in a large proportion of cases, but for individuals with a dual diagnosis, this categorization often excludes them from long-term care programs and services.

Most communities have agencies that help health care and social services professionals locate and gain access to long-term care services. These information and referral services can be found in local Area Agencies on Aging, Alzheimer's Association chapters, hospitals, and geriatric and mental health clinics. Case management services are also available, which help families navigate the health care and social services systems.

CONCLUSION

It is important to remember that most dementing illnesses are progressive degenerative diseases and that the needs of the person with dementia will change. It is not always possible for people with dementia to "age in place," and often it is necessary for families to seek alternative care options. New patterns of care are emerging that emphasize medical/psychiatric evaluations and behavior management, combined with mental health services, in long-term care facilities. Case management programs offer single-entry access to a variety of social, medical, ancillary, supportive, and concrete services that provide a continuum of care.

As the long-term care system has evolved, the number of options available to meet the needs of older people has increased. Providers and regulators need to examine the ways in which community programs and residential care settings serve people with dementia and work to ensure that the needs of older people with behavior disorders are being met in the long-term care system.

REFERENCES

Alzheimer's Association. (1994). *Residential settings: An examination of Alzheimer issues.* Chicago: Author.

Gerdner, L.A., & Buckwalter, K.C. (1996). Review of state policies regarding special care units: Implications for family consumers and health care professionals. *American Journal of Alzheimer's Disease, H*(2), 16–27.

Hutton, J.T., Dippel, R.L., Loewenson, R.B., Mortimer, J.A., & Christians, B.L. (1985). Predictors of nursing home placement of patients with Alzheimer's disease. *Texas Medicine, 81*, 40–43.

Joint Commission on Accreditation of Healthcare Organizations. (1996). *Comprehensive accreditation manual for long term care.* Chicago: Author.

Kaplan, M. (1996). Challenges to success. In S.B. Hoffman & M. Kaplan (Eds.), *Special care programs for people with dementia* (pp. 1–15). Baltimore: Health Professions Press.

Knopman, D.S., Kitto, J., Deinard, S., & Heiring, J. (1988). Longitudinal study of death and institutionalization in patients with primary degenerative dementia. *Journal of the American Geriatrics Society, 36*, 108–112.

Smallegan, M. (1985). There was nothing else to do: Needs for care before nursing home admission. *Gerontologist, 25*(4), 364–369.

U.S. Congress, Office of Technology Assessment. (1992). *Special care units for people with Alzheimer's and other dementias* (Report No. OTA-H-543). Washington, DC: U.S. Government Printing Office.

2

Innovations in
Behavior Management

Stephanie B. Hoffman, Ph.D.

Innovations in the behavior management of older adults with dementia are surprisingly rare. The primary reason for this is the continued reliance on a medical model for management (Garrard et al., 1991; Lantz et al., 1990). Hepburn, Severance, Gates, and Christensen (1989) found that medication and restraints are the most frequent responses to disruptive behaviors. In addition, isolating people with dementia on dementia-specific care units (DSCUs), difficulties in conducting research, and the pervading sense of helplessness and frustration felt by staff and family caregivers all contribute to a dearth of new treatments. What seems more essential than innovations is a concerted application of interventions that are already known to be effective.

INTERVENTIONS THAT STIMULATE THE SENSES

Because of their cognitive decline, people with Alzheimer's disease do not benefit from complex activities. Simple and enjoyable sensory stimulation programs are especially useful when working with older people with dementia. However, many of these older adults are isolated in small DSCUs, with little or no outside activities. Older adults experience sensory deprivation and isolation if a structured program of activities is not offered. Such a program requires activity staff who are trained in dementia care and are assigned to these older adults. Although volunteers may supplement staff, they must be trained carefully. Many books and chapters (see Chapters 9 and 10) address the activity needs of people with dementia; the only cautionary note is that these programs must indeed be carried out. In a 3-month observational study Cohen-Mansfield, Marx, and Werner (1992) found that residents were involved in no activities at all 63% of the time and in structured activities only 5% of the time. Additionally, residents were more agitated when unoccupied. Burnout, staff turnover, lack of administrative support, and floating staff make the implementation of structured activities precarious. Nursing staff also must make a commitment to ensuring that residents attend these programs, which is difficult when they have other pressing responsibilities.

The A.G.E. (Activities, Guidelines for Psychotropic Medications, and Education) program, developed and tested by Rovner, Steele, Shmuely, and Folstein (1996), demonstrated that a daily program of activities, a decrease in psychotropic drug use following careful guidelines, and educational rounds reviewing the residents had significant effects. As a result of the 6-month program, far fewer treatment group residents exhibited behavior problems, were on antipsychotic medications, or were restrained. The activity program consisted of a day program within the facility, which operated from 10:00 A.M. to 3:00 P.M. This program emphasized creative arts, music, exercise, and other activities described in *Doing Things* (Zgola, 1987). A psychiatrist tapered residents off psychotropic drugs and prescribed antidepressants as indicated. Educational rounds consisted of the psychiatrist's meeting weekly with the activities staff to discuss symptoms and their causes for each resident.

The newer interventions are those that consume little staff time. Snoezelen, described more fully in Chapter 11, is carried out in a room using a variety of gentle stimuli for all of the senses (see Figure 1). Residents can experience the sensations in the room with little staff interaction.

Another intervention, simulated presence therapy (SPT), utilizes the comforting voice of a loved one recorded on audiotape. According to Woods and Ashley (1995), "On the SPT audiotape, a caregiver 'converses' about cherished memories, loved ones, family anecdotes, and other best loved experiences of the patient's life" (p. 10). These tapes are edited carefully to include only those topics that the older person enjoys. The person wears headphones to listen to the tape, which is about 15 minutes long, and the tape can be played often (because the resident forgets hearing it). The SPT intervention was effective in treating social isolation, the most common behavior problem identified by nursing staff, as well as agitation.

Video Respite (Lund, Hill, Caserta, & Wright, 1995) is an innovative videotape intervention that is the basis for an emerging national research program that studies the effectiveness of specially developed video programming. The

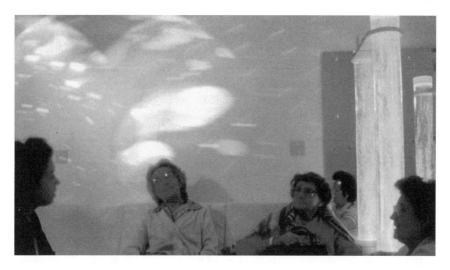

Figure 1.   Snoezelen therapy combines soft lighting, gentle music, tactile surfaces, and essential oils to stimulate the senses of older adults with dementia in a comfortable, safe environment. (Photograph courtesy of ROMPA® International, Chesterfield, England. sales@rompa.co.uk)

researchers have tested individual-specific video respite tapes that are similar to SPT audiotapes. Although caregivers found it somewhat burdensome or anxiety-provoking to have the videos prepared, they did use the tapes often and from them gained much-needed free time. The researchers then developed generic videos with titles such as "Gonna Do a Little Music," "Remembering When," and "A Visit with Maria" (in Spanish). Actors, who assume the role of visitors to the person with dementia, tell stories, sing, ask questions, smile, and encourage the older person to follow along. People with dementia seem to find the tapes enthralling and enjoyable. Behavior problems such as wandering, complaining, withdrawing, and asking repeated questions are reduced (tapes can be ordered from Innovative Caregiving Resources by calling 800-249-5600) (Angelleli, Lund, Pratt, & Hare, 1994).

VISUAL STIMULATION

Innovations in visual stimulation include environmental design by architects and interior designers specially trained in the intricacies of long-term care environments. Such experts recognize the need for visual contrast, adequate lighting, areas of natural light, incorporation of gardens and plants, and use of old-fashioned furniture and pictures. The placement of environmental features can either encourage or discourage activities of daily living (ADLs). Visible toilets placed in the center of the bedroom, such as those utilized at the Corinne Dolan Alzheimer

Care and Applied Research Center (Chardon, Ohio), support toileting activities in residents (Harr, 1995). The Americana Room at the Jewish Home of Central New York in Syracuse uses pictures of original magazine advertisements from the 1930s and 1940s and videotapes of classic movies (Bloodgood, 1995). The Arden Hill Life Care Center in Goshen, New York, incorporates indoor and outdoor gardens in resident treatment plans—a traveling garden on wheels is used for in-room visits (Gallivan & Hopkins, 1995).

Newspapers, magazines, and large-print books are familiar materials. Although people with dementia may not understand what they are looking at, they may still enjoy the familiar ritual of looking through printed materials.

Art therapy, utilizing paints, modeling clay, and other nontoxic media, encourages expression and enhances or builds self-esteem. Even coloring with crayons or markers, which awakens satisfying long-term memories, may be quite enjoyable. Completed pictures provide individuals with dementia with a sense of accomplishment.

Light can be used to regulate body rhythms and facilitate a lessening of depression, a widespread problem among older adults. Satlin, Volicer, Ross, Herz, and Campbell (1992) use a bright-light treatment program to encourage nighttime sleeping, which is often disturbed or otherwise affected by depression. This treatment program consists of a week of evening (7:00 P.M.–9:00 P.M.) exposure to 1,500–2,000 lux of fluorescent light-box light while seated in a geri-chair. Brawley (1997) suggests that high levels of illumination with careful attention to glare encourages a better quality of life in people with dementia (see Chapter 8 for details).

AUDITORY STIMULATION

Many older adults have hearing deficits. These deficits can lead to problems with understanding speech, pain as the result of a phenomenon known as *recruitment* (i.e., overarousal of sensory neurons), and withdrawal from social situations. Residents of nursing facilities are bombarded with auditory stimulation: alarms, call bells, carts wheeling down the hall, the sounds of care activities, echoing water noise in the bathrooms, constant yelling or moaning by other residents, staff discussion, discordant televisions and radios, and overhead announcements. The decibel level of this noise can rival that of a jet plane flying directly overhead (Sloane, 1997). The easiest intervention is to turn off alarms and televisions and replace this noise with more comforting sounds. Music therapy is covered in depth by Tabloski in Chapter 9.

Burgio, Scilley, Hardin, Hsu, and Yancey (1996) suggest that environmental white noise be used to decrease verbal agitation (e.g., screams, moans, curses, self-talk, repetition). They used two audiotapes, either the continuous sound of water rushing over rocks in a stream or the gentle sound of ocean waves (these tapes are inexpensive and available from The Nature Company, Berkeley, CA).

Nursing assistants were encouraged to use the audiotapes on residents who were predetermined by researchers to respond favorably to the intervention. Burgio et al. found that the use of white noise helped to reduce verbal agitation by 23%.

TACTILE STIMULATION

Touch is important at all ages, but particularly so with older adults, as their other senses diminish. However, tactile stimulation must be approached with caution, as it may be mistakenly perceived as sexual/inappropriate in nature. Also, people with dementia may have many areas of pain on their bodies that they cannot report because of communication difficulties. Touch may exacerbate the pain from fractures, contractures, muscles in spasm, and areas of skin breakdown.

Snyder, Egan, and Burns (1995) suggest that hand massage can produce relaxation and decrease agitated behaviors, such as grabbing, screaming, hitting, and wandering. However, it is not consistently effective in reducing the frequency and intensity of agitation during personal care. Hand massage was more effective in the female subjects studied than in the male subjects. Hand massage has varying protocols; for example, changing the pressure and direction of strokes to the back and palm of the older person's hand, finger massage, and enclosing the person's hand within the massager's. Staff must be taught how to administer massage appropriately and to take care with injured areas on the skin.

Tactile stimulation with objects provided by many rehabilitation companies is particularly useful.[1] Older adults seem drawn to textured materials, objects with beads, and soft materials (Mayers & Griffin, 1990). Cuddling with dolls and stuffed animals is also beneficial. Although some staff may feel that such objects infantilize residents, anecdotal evidence suggests that these items are a welcome addition. Vinyl fabrics, although water repellent, may feel uncomfortable and foreign to older adults. According to Brawley (Chapter 8), "Vinyl furniture and plastic-wrapped sofas and chairs are neither familiar nor friendly."

A therapy that is particularly appropriate for people with dementia is animal-assisted (pet) therapy. The cuddling and petting of pets, for individuals who enjoy animals, may encourage relaxation and decrease agitation (Mosher-Ashley & Barrett, 1997; Zisselman, Rovner, Shmuely, & Ferrie, 1996).

KINESTHETIC STIMULATION

In combination with appropriate music, exercise may provide physical and social benefits to people with dementia. Payten and Porter (1994) found that the Armchair Aerobics program was enjoyed by most of its participants. The use of

---

[1]For example, Geriatric Resources' catalog features items such as a pat mat, stuffed animals, puzzles, match-and-sort objects, and a discovery apron with attached keys. Call (505) 524-0250 to obtain a catalog.

colorful balls and scarves elicited positive responses from the program participants. Improvement was shown in socialization, attention, sleep, smiles, and eye
contact. However, the majority of participants did not improve in areas of aggression, wandering, or mood swings. Payten and Porter (1994) suggest using a circle format and slow, gentle, rhythmic exercises accompanied by big band music
from the 1920s and 1930s.

ORAL AND OLFACTORY STIMULATION

People with cognitive impairment may have little control over the foods they are
given to eat in a long-term care setting. In planning meals, facility staff should
keep in mind that enjoyment of food may be the last pleasure that residents have
left to them. Some older adults may show resistance to unfamiliar foods. Staff
should contact family members to discern residents' favorite foods. Because of
dysphagia (i.e., swallowing difficulties resulting from stroke or dementia), solid
foods may need to be puréed and liquids thickened. Regardless, these foods
should still be appealing through careful shaping and addition of condiments.
Older people should not be hurried through their meals.

To stimulate the olfactory sense, familiar, comforting aromas (e.g., cookies
baking, popcorn, flowers) should permeate a facility. A good way to bolster or
increase residents' self-esteem, as well as to stimulate their sense of smell, is for
them to prepare snacks, bake, or arrange fresh flowers.

INDIVIDUALIZED BEHAVIORAL TREATMENTS

Given that a dementing disease may result from multiple etiologies and that other
physical and psychiatric ailments may be comorbid, individualized behavioral
treatments are sensible. No single treatment succeeds with all people with
dementia.

Staff must be alert to specific interventions that seem to calm their particular residents. Some residents may be calmed by a combination of two seemingly
unlikely things, such as eating crackers while listening to music. Residents with
a religious past may be calmed by quotations from scripture or by discussions
with a chaplain. It is helpful to know the residents' past coping strategies, such as
going for long walks, reading light fiction, smoking, or talking with friends. These
activities may still be successful in promoting relaxation.

Mayers (1994) recommends relaxation procedures that can be conducted
easily with older adults. One such procedure is interactive guided imagery
(Rossman & Breslar, 1992), a self-soothing technique. The clinician first encourages the individual to breathe slowly for several minutes, repeating the instruction frequently in a soothing manner. The person is then encouraged to think of
a happy scene, which should be individualized based on family or resident inter-

view. Although the self-soothing technique has not been evaluated in people with dementia, it seems easy to implement and may be quite comforting.

A "CARE MAP" FOR MANAGING DISRUPTIVE BEHAVIORS

One of the most innovative approaches to behavior management is a "care map" developed by Williams, Wood, Moorleghen, and Chittuluru (1995), entitled the Disruptive Behavior Decision Model (DBDM). The DBDM uses four interventions:

- Optimal stimulation
- Problem ownership
- Environmental alteration
- Applied behavior analysis

Prior to the application of these interventions, medical reasons (e.g., pain, fatigue, infection, constipation, medication problems) causing the disruptive behavior must be ruled out. If these conditions are not the cause of the behavior disorder, stimulation issues—is there too much going on or not enough? Is the resident involved in the appropriate level of activities?—must be addressed (optimal stimulation). If stimulation issues are not the problem, then a decision must be made as to whether there is an actual problem (i.e., problem ownership)—is the behavior harmful to the resident or others? Is lack of training or understanding by staff causing the disruptive behavior? Perhaps the resident's environment is causing the behavior and an environmental alteration may change it. If a change in the environment does not improve the person's behavior, the most staff-intensive intervention—applied behavior analysis—should be implemented. In applied behavior analysis the target behavior must be identified. Then, behavioral antecedents and consequences are tracked; either or both can be changed, and the incidence of target behavior is then documented. Williams et al. use a decision tree, which can be the basis for staff training. The model has been evaluated only informally, but staff who have used it report less conflict and more creativity in behavior management.

RESOURCES FOR ENHANCING
ALZHEIMER'S CAREGIVER HEALTH (REACH) PROGRAM

The National Institute on Aging is funding several large research projects to develop and test new ways to help family and professional caregivers manage the stresses of caring for people with dementia. The coordinating center for the project is located at the University of Pittsburgh, in the offices of Dr. Richard Schulz. Outcomes from these projects should include some carefully evaluated interventions that will decrease behavior disruptions.

BEHAVIOR MANAGEMENT SKILLS

If used consistently, behavior management skills improve the effectiveness of staff in dealing with dementia-related behavior disorders. Stevens et al. (in press) developed a training program for nursing assistants that focuses on five skill areas:

- Identification of environmental factors affecting behavior
- Use of the ABC approach (antecedents-behaviors-consequences)
- Communication techniques
- Positive reinforcement
- Distraction/diversion strategies

On-the-job training and feedback are also provided to the adult learners by trainers. As part of this program, nursing assistants self-monitor their skills daily using a brief checklist. The checklist monitors the following 11 behaviors:

- Being in visual proximity to the resident before addressing him or her
- Greeting the resident by name during every caregiving session
- Identifying self to the resident before each caregiving session
- Giving verbal prompts
- Delaying by 5 seconds physical assistance after a verbal prompt
- Announcing each activity during a caregiving task
- Delaying by 5 seconds physical assistance after an announcement
- Giving one-step instructions
- Speaking slowly
- Praising independent ADLs
- Praising the resident for following instructions

Supervisors are also encouraged to monitor, via the Formal Staff Management system, implementation of these skills by nursing assistants in order to maintain their daily use through observation of nursing assistant performance and provision of positive/constructive feedback. Incentives are made possible, such as time off (leaving work 30 minutes early each day for a week) for 80% accuracy in using these skills. The Formal Staff Management system, according to Stevens et al. (in press), is a critical component of the program, and ensures that skills are implemented and maintained.

BEHAVIORAL INTENSIVE CARE UNIT

Mintzer and colleagues (1993) describe an inpatient behavioral intensive care unit (BICU), the goal of which is to develop treatment plans for people who are agitated and return them to the home setting. The home is modified, and primary caregivers are trained to carry out the necessary interventions. The three components of the BICU program are implemented, one per week, for a typical length of stay of 21 days.

Week 1 includes the identification and evaluation of target behaviors. Residents are monitored frequently (in some cases, every 30 minutes). An interdisciplinary team consisting of several physicians, a neurologist consultant, psychologist, pharmacist, social worker, advanced practice nurse, dietitian, occupational therapist, and recreation therapist meets daily to discuss these observations. During Week 2, the individualized treatment plan is implemented and adjusted. The focus of Week 3 is discharge planning: An occupational therapist conducts a home visit to evaluate whether the home can support the treatment plan. Primary caregivers are trained by all relevant staff, and a family discharge conference is conducted. A follow-up home visit by a registered nurse is conducted 1 week postdischarge to offer additional training and environmental modification.

In Mintzer et al.'s study, 75% of the residents were discharged home. At a 6-month follow-up, no participant had been readmitted to any institutional setting.

ENVIRONMENT–BEHAVIOR MODEL

Zeisel, Hyde, and Levkoff (1994) outline an environment–behavior (E–B) model that can influence the quality of life of residents of DSCUs. They suggest that such units should be rated based on the following characteristics: exit control, wandering paths, private spaces, common space structure, outdoor freedom, residential scale, autonomy support, and sensory comprehension. They have developed a checklist to evaluate DSCUs using these dimensions and have included a list of resident and staff outcome variables that indicate quality of life and therapeutic outcomes. The E–B model provides an excellent integration of research in the field; designers and DSCU staff should use it in developing or renovating both space and special care programs. A well-designed environment, coupled with a well-trained staff, are probably the best strategies available for managing the behavior disorders of people with dementia.

CONCLUSION

Many caregivers are trained in how to manage behavior disorders. However, much of this training is not practiced during daily care. Administration and supervisors must make an effort to support staff, reward their efforts, and allow for their creativity. Because dementia is the result of a variety of causes, many creative approaches may need to be attempted before a solution is found to a resident's perplexing behavior problem. Caregivers need the motivation to keep on trying. DSCUs need staff who are assigned specifically to the unit, an appropriate number of staff, a nurturing environment, ongoing training, and adequate activities programs. Such units will indeed encourage a climate of high morale and creative, innovative approaches to care.

REFERENCES

Angelleli, J., Lund, D.A., Pratt, C., & Hare, J. (1994). *Video Respite in special care units for persons with dementia: An evaluation of its use and effectiveness.* Final report to the University of Utah Gerontology Center and the Ben and Iris Margolis Charitable Foundation, Salt Lake City.

Bloodgood, M.E. (1995). *Americana therapy* (Abstract). Jewish Home of Central New York, 4101 East Genessee Street, Syracuse, NY 13214.

Brawley, E.C. (1997). *Designing for Alzheimer's disease: Strategies for better care environments.* New York: John Wiley & Sons.

Burgio, L., Scilley, K., Hardin, J.M., Hsu, C., & Yancey, J. (1996). Environmental "white noise": An intervention for verbally agitated nursing home residents. *Journal of Gerontology: Psychological Sciences, 51B*(6), 364–373.

Cohen-Mansfield, J., Marx, M.S., & Werner, P. (1992). Observational data on time use and behavior problems in the nursing home. *Journal of Applied Gerontology, 11*(1), 111–121.

Gallivan, M.J., & Hopkins, M.A. (1995). *Pianos, peaches, and pines: Peaceful partnerships and compassionate environments for residents with Alzheimer's disease and related disorders* (Abstract). Arden Hill Life Care Center, 6 Harriman Drive, Goshen, NY 10924.

Garrard, J., Makris, L., Dunham, T., et al. (1991). Evaluation of neuroleptic drug use by nursing home elderly under proposed Medicare and Medicaid regulations. *Journal of the American Medical Association, 265*, 463–467.

Harr, R.G. (1995). *Applied research designs that enhance the environmental and programmatic autonomy for those suffering from Alzheimer's disease* (Abstract). Heather Hill, 12340 Bass Lake Road, Chardon, OH 44204-9364.

Hepburn, K., Severance, J., Gates, B., & Christensen, M. (1989, March/April). Institutional care of dementia patients: A state-wide survey of long-term care facilities and special care units. *American Journal of Alzheimer's Care and Related Disorders and Research,* pp. 19–23.

Lantz, M., Louis, A., Lowenstein, G., et al. (1990). A longitudinal study of psychotropic prescriptions in a teaching nursing home. *American Journal of Psychiatry, 147*(12), 1637–1639.

Lund, D.A., Hill, R.D., Caserta, M.S., & Wright, S.D. (1995). Video Respite: An innovative resource for family, professional caregivers, and persons with dementia. *Gerontologist, 35*(5), 683–687.

Mayers, K.S. (1994, July/August). Calming the agitated demented patient: Use of self-soothing techniques. *American Journal of Alzheimer's Care and Related Disorders & Research,* pp. 2–5.

Mayers, K., & Griffin, M. (1990). The play project: Use of stimulus objects with demented patients. *Journal of Gerontological Nursing, 16*(1), 32–37.

Mintzer, J.E., Lewis, L., Pennypaker, L., Simpson, W., Bachman, D., Wohlreich, G., Meeks, A., Hunt, S., & Sampson, R. (1993). Behavioral Intensive Care Unit (BICU): A new concept in the management of acute agitated behavior in elderly demented patients. *Gerontologist, 33*(6), 801–806.

Mosher-Ashley, P.M., & Barrett, P.W. (1997). *A life worth living: Practical strategies for reducing depression in older adults* (pp. 144–165). Baltimore: Health Professions Press.

Payten, A., & Porter, V. (1994). Armchair aerobics for the cognitively impaired. *Activities, Adaptation & Aging, 18*(2), 27–39.

Rossman, M.L., & Breslar, D.E. (1992). *Interactive guided imagery: An intensive training program for clinicians.* Mill Valley, CA: Academy for Guided Imagery, Inc.

Rovner, B.W., Steele, C.D., Shmuely, Y., & Folstein, M.F. (1996). A randomized trial of dementia care in nursing homes. *Journal of the American Geriatrics Society, 44*, 7–13.

Satlin, A., Volicer, L., Ross, V., Herz, L., & Campbell, S. (1992). Bright light treatment of behavioral and sleep disturbances in patients with Alzheimer's disease. *American Journal of Psychiatry, 119*, 1028–1032.

Sloane, P. (1997, May). *Bathing and screaming.* Paper presented at the 3rd Biennial DSCU Conference, St. Petersburg, FL.

Snyder, M., Egan, E.C., & Burns, K.R. (1995). Efficacy of hand massage in decreasing agitation behaviors associated with care activities in persons with dementia. *Geriatric Nursing, 16*(2), 60–62.

Stevens, A., Burgio, L.D., Bailey, E., Burgio, K., Paul, P., Capilouto, E., Nicovich, P., & Hale, G. (in press). Teaching and maintaining behavior management skills with nursing assistants in a nursing home. *Gerontologist.*

Williams, D.P., Wood, E.C., Moorleghen, F., & Chittuluru, V.C. (1995). A decision model for guiding management of disruptive behaviors in demented residents of institutionalized settings. *American Journal of Alzheimer's Disease, 10*(3), 22–29.

Woods, P., & Ashley, J. (1995). Simulated Presence Therapy: Using selected memories to manage problem behaviors in Alzheimer's disease patients. *Geriatric Nursing, 16*(1), 9–14.

Zeisel, J., Hyde, J., & Levkoff, S. (1994, March/April). Best practices: An Environment–Behavior (E–B) model for Alzheimer special care units. *American Journal of Alzheimer's Care and Related Disorders & Research*, pp. 4–21.

Zgola, J.M. (1987). *Doing things: A guide to programming activities for persons with Alzheimer's disease and related disorders.* Baltimore: The Johns Hopkins University Press.

Zisselman, M.H., Rovner, B.W., Shmuely, Y., & Ferrie, P. (1996). A pet therapy intervention with geriatric psychiatry inpatients. *American Journal of Occupational Therapy, 50*(1), 47–51.

3

Assessing and Understanding Agitated Behaviors in Older Adults

Jiska Cohen-Mansfield, Ph.D., and Levi Taylor, Ph.D.

Dementia is a chronic, unremitting, progressive disease. Although memory loss is the most widely recognized concomitant of the organic brain deterioration featured in dementia, behavior problems result as well, and are commonly clustered under the label "agitation"; in fact, agitation is one of the most common reasons for nursing facility placement (Colerick & George, 1986). The disruption caused by agitation detracts directly from the quality of life of all residents of nursing facilities in several ways, such as by alarming or frightening them; by interfering with their activities; by invading their personal space via touching or even harming them; or by touching, damaging, or taking their possessions. In addition, agitation can diminish the quality of care residents of nursing facilities receive by forcing staff members to spend their time managing agitation instead of addressing other resident needs. Moreover, agitation increases staff members' occupational stress (Cohen-Mansfield, 1995), thereby increasing absenteeism and turnover. The person who is most victimized by agitation is, however, the person who manifests it: A display of agitated behavior sometimes leads to being physically restrained or being placed on debilitating psychotropic medication, and it often results in social isolation.

Specific types of agitated behavior tend to co-occur, forming a distinctive syndrome. Four of those syndromes have been identified (Cohen-Mansfield,

Marx, & Rosenthal, 1989; Cohen-Mansfield, Werner, Watson, & Pasis, 1995), with examples of behaviors:

- Physically nonaggressive behavior—Performing repetitious mannerisms, pacing, inappropriate handling of objects, aimless walking, inappropriate dressing or undressing
- Physically aggressive behavior—Hitting, pushing, scratching, kicking, grabbing objects, grabbing people
- Verbally nonaggressive behavior—Frequently requesting attention, bossiness or pushiness, complaints or whining, negativism, stubbornness, unnecessary interruptions
- Verbally aggressive behavior—Cursing, exhibiting temper outbursts, making strange or menacing noises, screaming

PREVALENCE

Several researchers have studied the prevalence of agitation among residents of nursing facilities and community-dwelling older adults and have obtained a wide range of results. For example, pacing/wandering behaviors have been reported to occur among as few as 3% of outpatients with a diagnosis of probable Alzheimer's disease (Reisberg, Borenstein, Salob, Franssen, & Georgeotas, 1987) to among as many as 59% in a study of both in- and outpatients diagnosed with dementia (Rabins, Mace, & Lucas, 1982). Noisy or disruptive verbal behaviors take place at rates ranging between 10% and 30% (Cariaga, Burgio, Flynn, & Martin, 1991; Ray, Taylor, Lichtenstein, & Meador, 1992), and the prevalence of aggressive behaviors in institutional settings ranges from 8% to 49% (Everitt, Fields, Sooumerai, & Avorn, 1991; Marx, Cohen-Mansfield, & Werner, 1990). The wide divergence in these results can be explained by the use of different populations as well as by different operationalized criteria in defining agitation, which partially accounts for why different methods, rating scales, and sources were used to study the prevalence of all types of agitation.

TIMING

A rather consistent pattern of occurrence of pacing/wandering activity was reported by Algase and Tsai (1991), who noted that it took place most frequently during the hours of 2 P.M.–4 P.M. and 6 P.M.–7 P.M. Cohen-Mansfield, Werner, Marx, and Freedman (1991) found that residents who paced did so at high levels throughout the day, except during mealtimes. In a study that involved questioning daytime staff members, Cariaga et al. (1991) found that verbal agitation is most likely to occur on awakening and before bathing or eating. In a different type of study involving around-the-clock observations, Cohen-Mansfield and Werner (1995) found that verbal agitation occurs most often during the evening and when residents are alone in their rooms at night. They also found that aggressive forms of agitation are more common at lunchtime, during the evening, and on cold nights.

CAUSES

To a casual observer, most agitated behaviors may appear to be "inappropriate" or "meaningless," when, in fact, many instances of agitation are an attempt by the individual with dementia to accommodate unmet needs, such as the need to communicate, the need to alleviate pain, or the need for social or tactile stimulation. In order to explore possible unmet needs, researchers have examined the antecedents and correlates of agitation, usually concentrating on health, psychological, or environmental factors.

HEALTH FACTORS

Physical discomfort or pain are health factors that are associated with some forms of agitation. Of particular concern is that agitation may result from an attempt to communicate discomfort under circumstances in which a person with severe cognitive impairment is no longer able to do so directly. For example, older adults who express their agitation by yelling or with negative vocalizations seem to experience a large number of medical conditions and high levels of pain (Cohen-Mansfield, Billig, Lipson, Rosenthal, & Pawlson, 1990).

The relationship between health status and physically aggressive behavior is less clear, although a positive association between aggressive behavior and urinary tract infections has been reported (Ryden & Bossenmaier, 1988). In contrast, people who engage in physically nonaggressive agitation have been reported to have fewer medical diagnoses than other individuals and better appetites (Cohen-Mansfield, Werner, et al., 1995). Some people who pace have akathisia (i.e., an inner sense of restlessness) due to neurodegenerative disease or to an adverse reaction to antipsychotic drugs or other medications (Mutch, 1992).

Some of the findings regarding health status and various types of agitation described here would be expected logically. For example, the fact that physically nonaggressive behaviors such as pacing/wandering tend to occur among people who are healthier may be partially due to the weakness concomitant with illness, which would prevent pacing/wandering. In addition, the strain and frustration inherent in illness or discomfort may reduce the ability to inhibit aggressive impulses, particularly among people with dementia.

PSYCHOLOGICAL FACTORS

A variety of psychological constructs have been related to agitation, including dementia, delusions and hallucinations, depression, premorbid personality, and sleep disturbances.

DEMENTIA

Cognitive impairment relates to all forms of agitation, although the relationship between agitation and stage of dementia varies across each syndrome (Cohen-Mansfield, Culpepper, & Werner, 1995; Cohen-Mansfield, Marx, & Rosenthal, 1990). For example, physically aggressive agitation is more likely to be manifested by individuals with severe cognitive impairment (Marx, Cohen-Mansfield, & Werner, 1990; Meddaugh, 1987; Nasman, Bucht, Eriksson, & Sandman, 1993; Patel & Hope, 1992; Ryden, 1988; Swearer, Drachman, O'Donnell, & Mitchell, 1988; Winger, Schirm, & Stewart, 1987). This relationship can be explained in at least two ways. For example, physical aggression may be due to the increased frustration that results from a person's decreased ability to communicate his or her needs, which, in turn, results in those needs remaining unmet more often. Alternatively, increased incidents of aggression among people with high levels of impairment could be the outcome of severe organic brain deterioration, resulting in behavioral disinhibition.

In contrast to findings with people who manifest aggressive behavior, certain types of verbally nonaggressive behavior such as complaining or requesting attention are associated with mild to moderate impairment (Cohen-Mansfield, Culpepper, & Werner, 1995; Cohen-Mansfield, Marx, & Rosenthal, 1990; Malone, Thompson, & Goodwin, 1993). This association is not surprising because some preservation of cognitive ability is necessary in order for a person to engage in verbal behaviors. As might be expected, other forms of agitated vocalizations, such as screaming or vocal outbursts, are associated with a greater degree of cognitive impairment (Reisberg, Franssen, Sclan, Kluger, & Ferris, 1989). Those behaviors are likely due to factors that are similar to those mentioned earlier regarding physical agitation, such as increased frustration because of increased impairment, or increased disinhibition resulting from advanced brain deterioration, as well as an attempt to communicate when a person's ability to do so effectively has deteriorated.

DELUSIONS/HALLUCINATIONS

It appears that experiences of delusions or hallucinations are related to most types of agitation. Delusions and hallucinations were found to be present significantly more often among individuals who engaged in both types of nonaggressive agitation than in people who did not manifest these types of agitation. A similar trend was found in the aggressive types (Cohen-Mansfield, Taylor, & Werner, in press). Hallucinations tended to occur frequently among agitated participants as well. These phenomena suggest that agitation and delusions/hallucinations interact, wherein the perceptual changes involved in delusions/hallucinations adversely affect mood, thereby increasing agitation. Similar findings were reported by other researchers (Deutsch, Bylsma, Rovner, Steele, & Folstein, 1991; Lachs, Becker, Siegal, Miller, & Tinetti, 1992; Steiger, Quinn, Toone, & Marsden, 1991).

DEPRESSION

Verbal agitation has been found to correlate with depressed affect, but similar results were not found with people who presented with physically nonaggressive or aggressive agitation (Marx & Cohen-Mansfield, 1988). It was suggested that depression was detected among people who were verbally agitated because those individuals were more cognitively intact than people who were physically agitated, and therefore better able to communicate their moods (e.g., via complaints or other negative comments) to caregivers. Older adults who displayed other forms of agitation were less able to communicate effectively because of their greater cognitive deficits, making it difficult for caregivers to detect mood changes among people manifesting physical types of agitation.

PREMORBID PERSONALITY

Personality traits before the onset of dementia relate positively to some forms of agitation. For example, caregivers of 58% of the participants in a community-based study perceived aggressive behavior to be an exaggeration of premorbid personality (Ware et al., 1990; see also Ryden, 1988). Similarly, individuals who pace or wander were reported to have been more active in premorbid life (Monsour & Robb, 1982), although subsequent research failed to replicate this finding (Cohen-Mansfield, Werner, Marx, & Freedman, 1991). Males are more likely than females to exhibit aggressive forms of agitation (Marx, Cohen-Mansfield, & Werner, 1990; Ryden & Bossenmaier, 1988), a phenomenon that corresponds to research (e.g., Krebs & Miller, 1985) that indicates that males are more likely than females to engage in physical aggression among the general population. Conversely, females are more likely than males to engage in verbally nonaggressive behavior, possibly reflecting consistent findings of greater verbal ability among females as compared with males among all age groups (Harasty, Double, Halliday, Krill, & McRitchie, 1997).

SLEEP DISTURBANCES

The impairment of circadian rhythms that is characteristic of Alzheimer's disease (e.g., Bliwise, 1993) is also related to agitation. In particular, an increase in agitation in older adults with dementia that occurs in the evening hours, beginning at a time near sunset, has been termed "sundowning." Disturbance in sleep patterns has been reported to relate to pacing or wandering, purposeless vocalizations, and verbal or physical aggression (Cohen-Mansfield & Marx, 1990).

ENVIRONMENTAL FACTORS

Environmental factors that have been found to be associated with verbally/vocally agitated behaviors include residents' being alone, being physically restrained, and being involved in an activity of daily living (ADL), especially toileting and bathing

(Cohen-Mansfield & Werner, 1995). Verbal agitation is more likely to occur in the evening hours. These data suggest that verbal agitation may be the result of an attempt to express an unmet social need, such as being alone and lonely, or a physical need, as may occur when the person is restrained.

In contrast to other agitated behaviors, wandering and pacing takes place under normal conditions of light, noise, and temperature, suggesting that these behaviors do not necessarily result from discomfort. Wandering and pacing occur most frequently in places, such as a corridor, lobby, or near the nurses' station, where other people are likely to be present (Cohen-Mansfield, Werner, et al., 1995), underscoring the notion that such behaviors may represent a person's attempt to increase his or her overall level of stimulation or activity.

Physically aggressive behaviors frequently take place in response to an intrusion into personal space by staff members or other residents (Bridges-Parlet, Knopman, & Thompson, 1994). In a study of environmental correlates of agitation, Cohen-Mansfield and Werner (1995) observed that aggressive behaviors occurred more often in social situations, when the temperature was cold, and when the individual was in close physical contact with another person, particularly staff members. It is probable that, in the presence of uncomfortable stimuli (e.g., ADLs, cold temperatures) or situations that are perceived to be threatening (e.g., invasion of personal space), individuals respond aggressively because of the deterioration of brain sites involved in the inhibition of aggressive behaviors or because of a limited repertoire of more appropriate responses.

SUMMARY: THEORETICAL UNDERPINNINGS

As the findings described here suggest, agitation results from an imbalance in the interaction among lifelong habits and personality, current physical and mental status, and less-than-optimal environmental conditions (see Figure 1). Most agitated behaviors arise because of dementia-related impairments in both communication and the ability to use the environment appropriately. These impairments cause frustration because they prevent the individual from meeting personal needs and because of the presence of the impairments themselves. Furthermore, in the presence of both frustration and organic brain deterioration, especially of the frontal lobe, disinhibition of the aggressive impulses that often are concomitant with frustration becomes more likely (Berkowitz, 1990). Some behaviors, such as trying to solicit help or self-stimulating, are instrumental, representing an effort to alleviate the need that triggered the behaviors.

ASSESSMENT

The care of older people is a duty shared by family members, physicians, and other health care professionals. In order to make responsible decisions regarding care regimens for each older adult reliable, relevant data regarding the individual's

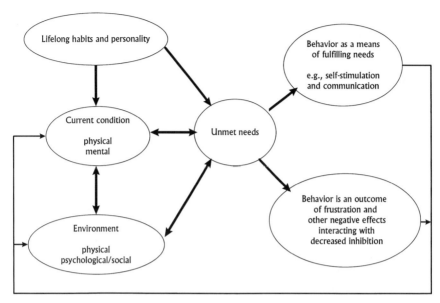

Figure 1.   Unmet needs model of agitated behavior.

condition must be collected. Because both the type of data sought and the method used to gather those data can affect the understanding of the scope of the problem, information regarding an older person's medical, cognitive, and behavioral status is required, as is information regarding the individual's functional status and the degree of familial and other types of support available to that person. For that reason a great many assessment instruments and assessment strategies have been developed for a wide variety of domains, including agitation and related constructs.

The assessment of agitation among older adults is complicated by the fact that most people who are agitated have dementia, which involves a progressive deterioration of language ability. As a result, asking people why they exhibit agitated behavior—the method that intuitively appears to be the most direct—almost always results in either an incomplete response or no coherent response at all. In order to address this problem a variety of strategies have been developed for measuring agitated behaviors. These strategies can be grouped into three general classes of approach: the use of observational methods, mechanical devices, and informant rating methods.

OBSERVATIONAL METHODS

Observational methods involve someone (usually research personnel) observing an individual and rating relevant behaviors as they occur. For example, a research assistant can be assigned to monitor the behavior of an older adult in his or her environment (e.g., a nursing facility). When a specific agitated behavior is observed, the assistant indicates that the event took place and then rates it along relevant dimensions such as duration, severity, and disruptiveness on a scale designed for that purpose. Alternatively, a mechanical device is sometimes used, wherein the research assistant presses a button on a handheld computer or scans a bar code from a list. This method has the advantage of providing a more exact measure of the duration of the observed behavior. Another technique is to video-tape the individual for a specified period of time in a relevant setting, and then ask a research assistant to watch the tape and rate the behavior. Videotaping is particularly useful for interrater reliability studies because two or more people can watch identical behaviors separately and at different times. It is also especially helpful when subtle behaviors are the focus of research because they can be watched several times and can be stopped and rewound. A drawback of observational methods for assessing agitation is that, because many types of agitation, especially physical aggression, do not occur most of the time, either extended periods of observation or many observation sessions are necessary to "capture" the behavior. Furthermore, thorough training of observers is essential for the ratings to be reliable.

An example of an instrument developed specifically for observing agitation is the Agitation Behavior Mapping Instrument (ABMI; Cohen-Mansfield, Werner, & Marx, 1989), which was developed in order to examine environmental correlates of agitation. The ABMI assesses several aspects of agitation, including the frequency of occurrence of the agitated behaviors, the social context in which the behavior took place, the type of activity engaged in when the behavior occurs, who initiated the activity, the location of the resident on the unit, environmental characteristics (e.g., light, noise), and the resident's body position.

MECHANICAL DEVICES

Mechanical devices can be used for assessing wandering behaviors. Two types of mechanism are used: instruments that gauge movement (e.g., actigraphs, personal activity monitors, large-scale activity monitors) and instruments that measure the number of steps taken (e.g., a pedometer or step sensor). The use of mechanical devices has the advantage of requiring less staff time for monitoring and, therefore, is less expensive generally than other measurement techniques. Furthermore, they are quite precise in their measurements (Cohen-Mansfield, Culpepper, Werner, Wolfson, & Bickel, 1997). A major drawback is that they can be used to measure only a very limited range of behavior.

INFORMANT RATING METHODS

A number of informant rating instruments have been developed for measuring agitation among older adults in the nursing facility and in the community. Many of these instruments include agitation or one of the subtypes of agitation as a dimension on a scale designed to measure other constructs as well. Others were designed to assess a particular subtype of agitation, usually aggression. Finally, some scales have been developed to measure agitation specifically and globally. Although it is not feasible to review all of the scales that measure some form of agitation among older people, the authors present examples of various informant rating scales in order to offer an overview of the range and diversity of approaches that have been employed in approaching the construct.

SCALES THAT INCLUDE MEASURES OF AGITATION IN ADDITION TO OTHER CONSTRUCTS

Several scales have been developed to measure behavioral and psychological changes that are concomitant with dementia that include measures of agitation. Some examples follow.

Behavioral Pathology in Alzheimer's Disease Rating Scale

One of the most commonly used caregiver-rated instruments is the Behavioral Pathology in Alzheimer's Disease Rating Scale (BEHAVE-AD; Reisberg et al., 1987), an instrument designed to measure behavioral problems and psychotic symptoms among outpatients of an aging and dementia research center. The BEHAVE-AD comprises 25 items, which are rated on a four-point Likert-type scale of severity, ranging from 0 = "not present" to 3 = "present generally with an emotional and physical component"; the BEHAVE-AD also contains a four-point global assessment of the magnitude of danger/disruptiveness of the behavior for both the person with dementia and his or her caregivers. The BEHAVE-AD was designed to measure the behavioral pathologies in dementia separately from cognitive and functional deficits with which they are associated (Reisberg, Auer, & Monteiro, 1996), and specifically taps seven separate categories of disturbance: paranoid/delusional ideation, hallucinations, activity disturbance (e.g., wandering, purposeless activity, inappropriate activity), aggressiveness, diurnal rhythm disturbance, affective disturbance, and anxieties and phobias.

Revised Memory and Behavioral Problems Checklist

The Revised Memory and Behavioral Problems Checklist (RMBPC; Teri et al., 1992) is a 24-item caregiver-rated inventory that assesses observable behavior problems among people with dementia. It uses a five-point Likert-type frequency scale, ranging from 0 = "never" to 4 = "daily or more often." In addition, it measures the degree to which the behaviors bothered or upset the caregiver also using a five-point Likert-type frequency scale, ranging from 0 = "not at all" to 4 = "extremely." The items for the RMBPC were derived both from possible items formulated by Teri and associates and from the original Memory and Behavioral Problems Checklist (MBPC; Zarit & Zarit, 1983), a caregiver-rated tool that assesses various behavior problems seen often among older people with dementia. Like the original MBPC, the RMBPC features three subscales that assess memory-related problems, depression problems, and disruption problems. The latter subscale, which is the most relevant to the study of agitation, assesses eight behaviors: arguing, waking up caregiver, being verbally aggressive, exhibiting embarrassing behavior, exhibiting dangerous behavior, talking loudly/rapidly, threatening to hurt others, and destroying property. The other subscales also contain items that are usually classified as agitation, such as repeating questions or hiding things. In addition to separate subscale scores for both the frequency of behavior problems and the degree of caregiver distress caused by the behavior, the RMBPC provides a total score for the two domains.

Neuropsychiatric Inventory

The Neuropsychiatric Inventory (NPI) was developed by Cummings, Mega, Gray, Rosenberg-Thompson, and Gornbein (1994) to assess simultaneously a wide range of behaviors exhibited by people with dementia, to provide a means of distinguishing between severity and frequency of the behavior changes, and to facilitate rapid assessment via the use of screening questions. Ten domains are evaluated by the NPI, including delusions/hallucinations, agitation/aggression, dysphoria, anxiety, apathy, disinhibition, irritability/lability, and aberrant motor activity. The NPI provides separate scores for both frequency and severity of each subscale, and a total score is calculated by multiplying frequency by severity.

Behavioral Syndromes Scale for Dementia

The Behavioral Syndromes Scale for Dementia (BSSD; Devanand et al., 1992) is a scale that focuses on agitation in considerable detail. Like other scales reviewed in this section, it measures behavioral syndromes that are concomitant with dementia. Specifically, the syndromes assessed by the BSSD are disinhibition (e.g., various types of physical aggression, verbal aggression, motor agitation), apathy/indifference, sundowning, denial, catastrophic reaction (e.g., anxiety, tears), and other clinical features (e.g., activities of daily living, emotional dependency, paranoia, stubbornness). Almost all of the items are rated on a seven-point Likert-type scale, ranging from 0 = "none" to 6 = "extreme," with the exception of "denial," which is rated on a four-point scale. All items are rated relative to the premorbid rate of manifestation of these behaviors. The caregiver who provides the information for the BSSD is specifically asked by the interviewer to base all responses primarily on observed behavior rather than on what is inferred.

SCALES DESIGNED TO MEASURE SPECIFIC TYPES OF AGITATION

Some forms of agitation are more disruptive and pose more of a threat than others. The most disruptive of these forms is aggression. Accordingly, several scales have been developed for the measurement of aggression.

Rating Scale for Aggressive Behaviour in the Elderly

The Rating Scale for Aggressive Behaviour in the Elderly (RAGE; Patel & Hope, 1992) is a 21-item checklist that measures aggressive behavior among psychogeriatric inpatients and is rated by nursing staff. Seventeen items assess specific types of aggressive behavior and are rated in a Likert-type format, ranging from 0 = "the behavior never occurs" to 3 = "the behavior occurred more than once in the past 3 days." Three questions are posed with regard to the consequences of the behavior, and the final item requires a global rating of the person's aggressiveness via a four-point scale.

Ryden Aggression Scale

The Ryden Aggression Scale (RAS; Ryden, 1988) characterizes the nature and frequency of the occurrence of aggressive behaviors among older adults. It is a 25-item Likert-type scale in which 0 = "the behavior never occurs" and 5 = "the behavior occurs once or more daily." It is a retrospective instrument that can be rated by family members or other caregivers and consists of three subscales, Physically Aggressive Behavior, Verbally Aggressive Behavior, and Sexually Aggressive Behavior.

Staff Observation Aggression Scale

Another scale designed for use among psychogeriatric inpatients is the Staff Observation Aggression Scale (SOAS; Palmstierna & Wistedt, 1987). The SOAS assesses both the nature and frequency of aggressive behaviors. The report form consists of five sections that require the rater to evaluate the nature of the provocation, the means used by the patient (e.g., verbal, hand, foot), the aim of aggression, the consequences for the object of the aggression, and the means used to end the aggression.

SCALES DESIGNED TO MEASURE AGITATION GLOBALLY

As examined earlier in the chapter, agitation features several components. Therefore, it should not seem surprising that a number of scales have been designed specifically to measure those components. In this section, two examples of agitation scales are presented: the Pittsburgh Agitation Scale and the Cohen-Mansfield Agitation Inventory.

Pittsburgh Agitation Scale

The Pittsburgh Agitation Scale (PAS; Rosen, Burgio, Kollar, et al., 1994) is a short rating scale for agitation that categorizes agitation into four items, "aberrant vocalization," "motor agitation," "aggressiveness," and "resisting care," which are rated on a four-point Likert-type scale of intensity.

Cohen-Mansfield Agitation Inventory

The Cohen-Mansfield Agitation Inventory (CMAI; Cohen-Mansfield, Marx, & Rosenthal, 1989; see Appendix) was developed originally for use in nursing facilities. Subsequently, a separate version was developed that can be used with older adults living in the community. The CMAI was created originally for research purposes. However, it has also been used for clinical purposes, such as determining whether withdrawal of psychotropic medication results in an increase in agitation. It is used by family caregivers, social workers, activity directors of adult day centers, nursing and social work staff in nursing facilities, and others.

The CMAI rates how often an older person exhibited 29 agitated behaviors within the past 2 weeks, using a Likert-type frequency scale ranging from 1 = "never" to 7 = "several times an hour." Examples of these behaviors include pacing/wandering, inappropriate robing or disrobing, complaining, cursing/verbal aggression, hurting self or others, and handling objects inappropriately. Each item measured by the CMAI actually captures a group of related behaviors. Because it is impossible to include all behaviors on the list, if the person to be rated manifests an inappropriate behavior that is close to a behavior on the CMAI, it can be subsumed under that category. An extended version of the CMAI includes measures of both the frequency and the perceived disruptiveness of each behavior, in which disruptiveness is rated on a five-point scale ranging from 1 = "not at all" to 5 = "extremely." The CMAI provides four scores, which correspond to the four types of agitated behaviors described in the introduction to the chapter.

SUMMARY: INFORMANT RATING INSTRUMENTS

Although the available informant rating instruments share similar items, they differ in many ways. Most fundamental, the constructs that are targeted are often dissimilar. One basic reason for this dissimilarity is that, when compiling their assessments, the various authors of agitation scales have assumed different, although often overlapping, definitions of agitation. For example, whereas the PAS and CMAI both feature four subscales of agitation, these subscales are not the same. Because of the different definitions of agitation, some scales have more clinical utility than others, whereas others provide more information that might be useful from a researcher's point of view.

Another difference among instruments concerns the identity of the informant used (i.e., family members, nursing assistants, charge nurses, physicians). Because of family members' close relationship to their loved one, they are often the best source of report for older adults living in the community. Nevertheless, family members' ratings can be skewed by their previous relationship with the person with dementia, by the strain imposed on them by caring for the older person, and by the extent of their understanding of the nature of the rating instruments.

Ratings provided by clinical staff such as nursing staff or physicians provide the benefit of being completed by professionals who are both educated and experienced in the use of assessment tools. The drawback of ratings provided by the latter group is that most assessments concern frequencies of behavior. However, the amount of contact between the informant and the older adult is at least limited to the shift on which the informant works, and, in the case of physicians, it can be limited to a few brief examination periods. Furthermore, as with family members, staff ratings can be influenced by their level of stress, job overload, or habituation to the behavior as a result of repeated exposure. In addition, both family and staff members may underreport behavior because they fear that an indication of frequent inappropriate behavior will reflect negatively either on the quality of care they provide or on the older adult. This underscores the need to emphasize to caregivers that behaviors in dementia are the result of an organic disease process and should be taken to reflect neither on the older person nor on the caregivers. The identity of the individual who completes the questionnaire is therefore an operative factor in the reliability of the assessment process.

Finally, it should be apparent that the construction and properties of the assessments differ. For example, some scales use a simple checklist format in which a behavior is marked as either "present" or "absent," whereas most scales use a Likert-type format. The dimension of the behavior that is scored also varies across the scales, in which most measure frequency, although some measure severity or disruptive impact. Similarly, the method of scoring differs, whereby straightforward measures of frequency, severity, or disruptiveness are most commonly computed, although frequency weighted by disruptive impact or severity is also sometimes used. In addition, the most frequently occurring, the most severe, or the most disruptive behavior receives special attention on some scales. Furthermore, some instruments provide a single score, some provide scores only for subscales or syndromes, and some provide both subscale and total scores. Naturally, differences in scoring procedures yield different results, and one's selection of a particular tool should therefore depend on one's purpose for using it.

SELECTION OF ASSESSMENT STRATEGY

A decision regarding whether to employ an observational method, an informant rating, or a mechanical device to assess agitation obviously depends primarily on one's purpose for performing the evaluation. In making a decision it is essential to consider 1) differences between the length of time involved in sampling, 2) varying degrees of objectivity across methodologies, and 3) differences in cost across the methods. For example, the length of time that can be assessed by informant ratings is considerably longer than by other methods because those instruments can retrospectively examine a rather long period of time, such as the previous 2 weeks or 1 month. Moreover, in contrast to other methods, informant ratings are usually less expensive. Because they rely on subjective judgments, however, informant ratings do not permit as precise a documentation of behavior as is sometimes needed.

Direct observations and videotapes cover a much narrower period of time. However, they expedite relatively close scrutiny of the agitated behavior, and in the case of videotapes they can be reviewed as many times as desired. Nevertheless, they require a substantial amount of observer time and therefore can be rather expensive. Mechanical devices can be used over longer periods of time and are precise; unfortunately, as already noted, there are few agitated behaviors that can be measured with them. As the preceding text suggests, some behaviors cannot be measured easily using certain strategies. For example, if a behavior occurs with low frequency, observational methods are impractical. In contrast, if an extremely subtle behavior that might not otherwise be detected is the focus, observational methods are usually better than other strategies.

CONCLUSION

Agitation is a complex phenomenon involving several subtypes. Although agitation is related to dementia, it is not fully explained by the presence of dementia because not every person with dementia exhibits agitation. Instead, a variety of other factors that are roughly subsumed under the domains of health, psychological, and environmental factors influence the manifestation of agitation. In general, agitated behaviors appear to be the outcome of an attempt to fulfill an unmet need in one of those domains, such as the need for stimulation or the need to alleviate discomfort. A variety of approaches have been established as effective in assessing agitation. Knowledge concerning the etiology and assessment of agitation provides a promising basis for better detection and treatment of this phenomenon in the future.

REFERENCES

Algase, D., & Tsai, J. (1991). Wandering as a rhythm. *Gerontologist, 31*(Program Abstracts), 140.

Bliwise, D. (1993). Sleep in normal aging and dementia. *Sleep, 16*(1), 40–81.

Bridges-Parlet, S., Knopman, D., & Thompson, T. (1994). A descriptive study of physically aggressive behavior in dementia by direct observation. *Journal of the American Geriatrics Society, 42*, 192–197.

Cariaga, J., Burgio, L., Flynn, W., & Martin, D. (1991). A controlled study of disruptive vocalizations among geriatric residents in nursing homes. *Journal of the American Geriatrics Society, 39*, 501–507.

Cohen-Mansfield, J. (1995). Stress in nursing home staff: A review and theoretical model. *Journal of Applied Gerontology, 14*, 444–446.

Cohen-Mansfield, J., Billig, N., Lipson, S., Rosenthal, A., & Pawlson, L. (1990). Medical correlates of agitated behaviors in nursing home residents. *Gerontology, 36*(3), 150–158.

Cohen-Mansfield, J., Culpepper, W.J., & Werner, P. (1995). The relationship between cognitive function and agitation in senior daycare participants. *International Journal of Geriatric Psychiatry, 3*(9), 217–225.

Cohen-Mansfield, J., Culpepper, W.J., Werner, P., Wolfson, M., & Bickel, E. (1997). Assessment of ambulatory behavior in nursing home residents who pace or wander: A comparison of four commercially available devices. *Dementia and Geriatric Cognitive Disorders, 8,* 359–365.

Cohen-Mansfield, J., & Deutsch, L. (1996). Agitation: Subtypes and their mechanisms. *Seminars in Clinical Neuropsychiatry, 1,* 325–339.

Cohen-Mansfield, J., & Marx, M.S. (1988). Relationship between depression and agitation in nursing home residents. *Comparative Gerontological Behavior, 2,* 141–146.

Cohen-Mansfield, J., & Marx, M. (1990). The relationship between sleep disturbances and agitation in a nursing home. *Journal of Aging and Health, 2*(1), 153–165.

Cohen-Mansfield, J., Marx, M.S., & Rosenthal, A.S. (1989). A description of agitation in a nursing home. *Journal of Gerontology: Medical Sciences, 44*(3), M77–M84.

Cohen-Mansfield, J., Marx, M.S., & Rosenthal, A.S. (1990). Dementia and agitation in nursing home residents: How are they related? *Psychology and Aging, 5*(1), 3–8.

Cohen-Mansfield, J., Marx, M., Werner, P., & Freedman, L. (1992). Temporal patterns of agitated nursing home residents. *International Psychogeriatrics, 4,* 197–206.

Cohen-Mansfield, J., Taylor, L., & Werner, P. (1998). Delusions and hallucinations in an adult daycare population: A longitudinal study. *American Journal of Geriatric Psychiatry, 6*(2), 104–121.

Cohen-Mansfield, J., & Werner, P. (1995). Environmental influences on agitation: An integrative summary of an observational study. *American Journal of Alzheimer's Care and Related Disorders & Research, 10*(1), 32–39.

Cohen-Mansfield, J., Werner, P., & Marx, M.S. (1989). An observational study of agitation in a nursing home. *Journal of Gerontology, 44,* M77–M84.

Cohen-Mansfield, J., Werner, P., Marx, M., & Freedman, L. (1991). Two studies of pacing in the nursing home. *Journal of Gerontology: Medical Sciences, 46,* M77–M83.

Cohen-Mansfield, J., Werner, P., Watson, V., & Pasis, S. (1995). Agitation in participants of adult day care centers: The experiences of relatives and staff members. *International Psychogeriatrics, 7*(3), 447–458.

Colerick, E., & George, L. (1986). Predictors of institutionalization among caregivers of Alzheimer's patients. *Journal of the American Geriatrics Society, 34,* 493–498.

Cummings, J.L., Mega, M., Gray, K., Rosenberg-Thompson, S., & Gornbein, T. (1994). The Neuropsychiatric Inventory: Comprehensive assessment of psychopathology in dementia. *Neurology, 44,* 2308–2314.

Deutsch, L.H., Bylsma, F.W., Rovner, B.W., Steele, C., & Folstein, M.F. (1991). Psychosis and physical aggression in probable Alzheimer's disease. *American Journal of Psychiatry, 148*(9), 1159–1163.

Devanand, D., Brockington, C., Moody, B., Brown, R., Mayeaux, R., Endicott, J., et al. (1992). Behavioral syndromes in Alzheimer's disease. *International Psychogeriatrics, 4* (Suppl. 2), 161–184.

Everitt, D., Fields, D., Sooumerai, S., & Avorn, S. (1991). Resident's behavior and staff distress in the nursing home. *Journal of the American Gerontological Society, 39,* 791–798.

Harasty, J., Double, K., Halliday, G.M., Krill, J., & McRitchie, D. (1997). Language-associated cortical regions are proportionally larger in the female brain. *Archives of Neurology, 54,* 171–176.

Krebs, D., & Miller, D. (1985). Altruism and aggression. In G. Lindzey & E. Aronson (Eds.), *Handbook of social psychology*. New York: Random House.

Lachs, M.S., Becker, M., Siegal, A.P., Miller, R.P., & Tinetti, M.E. (1992). Delusions and behavioral disturbances in cognitively impaired elderly persons. *Journal of the American Gerontological Society, 40*, 768–773.

Malone, M.L., Thompson, L., & Goodwin, J.S. (1993). Aggressive behavior among institutionalized elderly. *Journal of the American Geriatrics Society, 41*, 853–856.

Marx, M., & Cohen-Mansfield, J. (1988). Relationship between depression and agitation in nursing home residents. *Comprehensive Gerontological Behavior, 2*, 141–146.

Marx, M., Cohen-Mansfield, J., & Werner, P. (1990). A profile of the aggressive nursing home resident. *Behavior, Health and Aging, 1*, 65–73.

Meddaugh, D.I. (1987). Aggressive and nonaggressive nursing home patients. *Gerontologist, 27*(Special Issue), 127A.

Monsour, N., & Robb, S.S. (1982). Wandering behavior in old age: A psychosocial study. *Social Work, 27*(5), 411–416.

Mutch, W.J. (1992). Parkinsonism and other movement disorders. In J.C. Brocklehurst, R.C. Tallis, & H.M. Fillit (Eds.), *Textbook of geriatric medicine and gerontology* (pp. 423). Edinburgh: Churchill Livingstone.

Nasman, B., Bucht, G., Eriksson, S., & Sandman, P.O. (1993). Behavioral symptoms in the institutionalized elderly—Relationship to dementia. *International Journal of Geriatric Psychiatry, 8*, 843–849.

Palmstierna, T., & Wistedt, B. (1987). Staff observation scale, SOAS: Presentation and evaluation. *Acta Psychiatrica Scandinavica, 76*, 657–663.

Patel, V., & Hope, R.A. (1992). Aggressive behavior in elderly psychiatric inpatients. *Acta Psychiatrica Scandinavica, 85*(2), 131–135.

Rabins, P.V., Mace, N.L., & Lucas, M.J. (1982). The impact of dementia on the family. *Journal of the American Medical Association, 248*, 333–335.

Ray, W., Taylor, J., Lichtenstein, M., & Meador, K. (1992). The nursing home behavior problem scale. *Journal of Gerontology, 47*, M9–M16.

Reisberg, B., Auer, S., & Monteiro, I. (1996). Behavioral pathology in Alzheimer's Disease Rating Scale. *International Psychogeriatrics, 8*(Suppl. 3), 301–308.

Reisberg, B., Borenstein, J., Salob, S., Franssen, E., & Georgeotas, A. (1987). Behavior symptoms in Alzheimer's disease. Phenomenology and treatment. *Journal of Clinical Psychiatry, 48*(5), 9–15.

Reisberg, B., Franssen, E., Sclan, S.G., Kluger, A., & Ferris, S.H. (1989). Stage specific incidence of potentially remediable behavioral symptoms in aging and Alzheimer's disease. *Bulletin of Clinical Neurosciences, 54*, 95–112.

Rosen, J., Burgio, L., Kollar, M., Cain, M., Allison, R., Fogelman, M., et al. (1994). The Pittsburgh Agitation Scale: A user-friendly instrument for rating agitation in dementia patients. *American Journal of Geriatric Psychiatry, 2*(1), 52–59.

Ryden, M.B. (1988). Aggressive behavior in persons with dementia living in the community. *Alzheimer Disease and Associated Disorders: International Journal, 2*(4), 342–355.

Ryden, M., & Bossenmaier, M. (1988). Aggressive behavior in cognitively impaired nursing home residents. *Gerontologist, 28*(Special Issue), 179A.

Steiger, M.J., Quinn, N.P., Toone, B., & Marsden, C.D. (1991). Off-period screaming accompanying motor fluctuations in Parkinson's disease. *Movement Disorders, 6*(1), 89–90.

Swearer, J.M., Drachman, D.A., O'Donnell, B.F., & Mitchell, A.L. (1988). Troublesome and disruptive behaviors in dementia: Relationships to diagnosis and disease severity. *Journal of the American Geriatrics Society, 36,* 784–790.

Teri, L., Truax, P., Logsdon, R., Uomoto, J., Zarit, S., & Vitaliano, P. (1992). Assessment of behavioral problems in dementia: The Revised Memory and Behavior Problems Checklist. *Psychology and Aging, 7,* 622–631.

Ware, C., Fairburn, C., & Hope, R. (1990). A community based study of aggressive behavior in dementia. *International Journal of Geriatric Psychiatry, 5,* 337–342.

Winger, J., Schirm, V., & Stewart, D. (1987). Aggressive behavior in long-term care. *Journal of Psychosocial Nursing, 25*(4), 28–33.

Zarit, S., & Zarit, J. (1983). Cognitive impairment. In P. Lewinson & L. Teri (Eds.), *Clinical geropsychology* (pp. 38–81). Elmsford, NY: Pergamon.

APPENDIX

THE COHEN-MANSFIELD AGITATION INVENTORY—LONG FORM

With Expanded Descriptions of Behaviors

Instructions:
Rate behaviors during past two weeks as they occurred on your shift. If prevented part of the time, estimate how frequently it would happen if not prevented. Do not include rare behaviors that are explained clearly by situational factors.

Rating scale for agitated behaviors

1—Never
2—Less than once a week
3—Once or twice a week
4—Several times a week
5—Once or twice a day
6—Several times a day
7—Several times an hour
8—Would be occurring if not prevented (e.g., would pace if not restrained)
9—Not applicable (e.g., cannot pace because cannot walk or move wheelchair)

1. **Pacing and aimless wandering**—Constantly walking back and forth; not indicating normal purposeful walk; including wandering when done in a wheelchair _____

2. **Inappropriate dressing or disrobing**—Putting on too many clothes, putting on clothing in a strange manner (e.g., putting pants on head), taking off clothing in public or when it is inappropriate (if only genitals are exposed, do not rate; see Item 28); do not rate person's ability to dress/undress as in ADLs _____

3. **Spitting (including while feeding)**—Spitting onto floor, other people, etc.; do not include salivating over which person has no control or spitting into tissue, toilet, or on ground outside _____

4. **Cursing or verbal aggression**—Only when using words; using obscenities, profanity, unkind speech or criticism, verbal anger, verbal combativeness (for nonverbal aggression, see Item 13) _____

5. **Constant unwarranted request for attention or help**—Verbal or nonverbal unreasonable nagging, pleading, demanding (indicate also for oriented people) _____

6. **Repetitive sentences or questions**—Repeating the same sentence or question one right after the other (do not include complaining—see Item 18; even if oriented and even if possibly warranted) _____

7. **Hitting (including self)**—Physical abuse, striking others, pinching others, banging self/furniture _____

8. **Kicking**—Strike people or objects forcefully using feet _____

9. **Grabbing onto people or objects inappropriately**—Snatching, seizing roughly, taking firmly, or yanking _____

10. **Pushing**—Forcefully thrusting, shoving, moving, putting pressure against _____

11. **Throwing objects**—Hurling, violently tossing up in air, tipping off surfaces, flinging, spilling food _____

12. **Making strange noises**—Crying, moaning, laughing weirdly, grinding teeth _____

13. **Screaming**—loud, shrill shouting; piercing howl _____

14. **Biting**—Chomp, gnash, gnaw (people or self) _____

15. **Scratching**—Clawing, scraping with fingernails (people or self) _____

16. **Trying to get to a different place**—Trying to leave the building, property; sneaking out of room; leaving inappropriately; trying to get into locked areas; trespassing within unit, into offices, other resident's room or closet _____

17. **Intentional falling**—Purposefully falling onto floor (includes from wheelchair, chair, or bed) _____

18. **Complaining**—Whining, complaining about self, making somatic complaints, griping (personal), complaining about external things or other people _____

19. **Negativism**—Bad attitude, does not like anything, nothing is right _____

20. **Eating or drinking inappropriate substances**—Putting into mouth and trying to swallow items that are inappropriate _____

21. **Hurting self or others**—Burning self or others, cutting self or others, touching self or others with harmful objects _____

22. **Handling things inappropriately**—Picking up objects that do not belong to them, rummaging through drawers, moving furniture, playing with food, fecal smearing _____

23. **Hiding things**—Putting objects under or behind something   ____

24. **Hoarding things**—Putting many or inappropriate objects in purse or pockets, keeping too many of one item   ____

25. **Tearing things or destroying property**—Shredding, ripping, breaking, stomping   ____

26. **Performing mannerisms repetitively**—Stereotypic movement, such as patting, tapping, rocking self; fiddling with something; twiddling something; rubbing self or object; sucking fingers; taking shoes on and off; picking at self, clothing, or objects; picking imaginary things out of air or off floor; manipulating nearby objects in a repetitious manner   ____

27. **Making verbal sexual advances**—Sexual propositions, sexual innuendo, or "dirty" talk   ____

28. **Making physical sexual advances or exposing genitals**—Touching a person in an inappropriate, sexual way; rubbing genital area; inappropriate masturbation, when not alone in own room or bathroom, unwanted fondling or kissing   ____

29. **General restlessness**—Fidgeting, getting up and sitting down (inability to sit still)   ____

For instructions concerning the administration and scoring of the CMAI, consult the CMAI manual.

II

Staff Roles in Caregiving

4

Training Staff in Behavior Management

Mary Kaplan, M.S.W., L.C.S.W., A.C.S.W.

Training of direct care staff in most long-term care facilities is focused on orientation to the facility, employee policies and procedures, specific care responsibilities, and basic skills. Minimal, if any, training is provided on the behavioral issues of residents with cognitive impairment. The behavior problems that are often seen in older adults with dementia may hinder the provision of care. Studies indicate that much of the physical and verbal aggression directed at staff by residents with dementia takes place during assistance with personal care (Bridges-Parlet, Knopman, & Thompson, 1994; Dougherty, Bolger, Preston, Jones, & Payne, 1992; Maxfield, Lewis, & Cannon, 1996). These behaviors are primarily an attempt by residents with dementia to communicate basic needs and concerns. Hindered and frustrated by the inability to express themselves clearly due to cognitive and language impairments, people with dementia often resort to a primitive means of communicating such as screaming and hitting.

It is essential that staff who work with people with dementia possess a basic understanding of the disease process as well as comprehend how cognitive losses affect behavior. It is important that training programs for any staff members who interact with residents with dementia include instruction in this area of dementia care in order to prevent or decrease problem behaviors. Research examining the effects of staff training on residents' behaviors suggests that there is evidence of reduction in the prevalence and/or the severity of behavioral disorders and an increase in appropriate behaviors following training (Austrom, 1996; Feldt & Ryden, 1992; Maxfield et al., 1996; Mentes & Ferrario, 1989).

Very few states have standards and regulations that mandate formal training programs for staff that care for people with dementia. As of 1996 five states (Iowa, Texas, Washington, Tennessee, and New Jersey) had adopted special regulations for dementia-specific care units (DSCUs; Gerdner & Buckwalter, 1996). Texas, Iowa, Tennessee, and New Jersey require the inclusion of behavior management in the training curriculum. However, these states vary in the minimum number of hours required for training, the types of staff that must be trained, and the minimum hours of annual continuing education required.

At the federal level, the Omnibus Budget Reconciliation Act of 1987 (OBRA '87) states that training programs for new nursing assistants working in long-term care facilities must include some training in the care of people with dementia. However, OBRA '87 regulations do not specify the amount of time or the type of information to be provided for training.

RELATIONSHIP BETWEEN TRAINING AND STAFF MORALE AND RETENTION

Without knowledge of the common behaviors manifested by people with dementia and strategies to successfully manage these behaviors, staff can quickly become frustrated and discouraged. The negative effects of this stress include emotional exhaustion, decreased feelings of personal achievement, and increased resentment toward and detachment from residents. If allowed to continue, a negative emotional state can lead to burnout, influencing organizational commitment, job satisfaction, and job retention (Henderson, 1987; Jayaratne & Chess, 1986; Kaplan, 1996b; Leiter & Maslach, 1988; Mobily, Maas, Buckwalter, & Kelly, 1992; Novak & Chappell, 1994; Peppard, 1986).

Although the time and resources required to train staff in dementia care are considerable, the effort can result in increased staff morale, improved teamwork, and decreased staff turnover (Austrom, 1996; Vance & Davidhizar, 1997). Training staff in the use of effective behavior management strategies provides them with alternatives to physical and chemical restraints. It also empowers them to handle challenging situations in ways that increase their sense of personal achievement and self-esteem, in addition to decrease stress and dysfunction in people with dementia. Appropriate responses to resident behaviors may help reduce burnout and lead to greater job satisfaction.

STAFF TRAINING

All staff training should be preceded by an assessment of the residents to determine their care needs and behaviors. This important first step enables trainers to design a program that includes strategies specific to the residents of the facility. It also provides baseline information with which to measure changes in resident behaviors and staff approaches posttraining. In order for staff training to succeed it must receive the full support of program administrators and managers. This support is essential when scheduling adjustments become necessary to allow staff to attend training sessions without jeopardizing staff coverage on the DSCU. Arrangements also should be made for staff to receive compensation for the time spent in training. In addition to providing the opportunity for staff training in dementia care, program administrators and department managers should receive training in the philosophy and elements of the dementia program (Kaplan, 1996a). Understanding the types of approaches and individualized care that are necessary for people with dementia enables management to support the efforts of the dementia care team by providing adequate staffing levels and developing job descriptions that allow for creative, nontraditional staff approaches.

Training in managing behaviors in dementia should not be limited to nursing staff. All employees—including housekeeping and dietary staff, rehabilitation therapists, activity therapists, social workers, and office staff (Kaplan, 1996a)—who interact with people with dementia need a basic knowledge of dementing illnesses, an understanding of the philosophy of the dementia program, and the ability to use appropriate communication skills and behavior management techniques. A key employee who is often overlooked in dementia care training is the receptionist, who sits at the entrance to the facility. In many cases she is the only person between the exit and the street when a resident with dementia wanders away from a secured area. Knowing about the behaviors of residents with dementia and ways to effectively redirect the residents may enable the receptionist to prevent them from leaving the building until other staff members can be summoned to provide assistance.

Some instruction in behavior management is included in the curriculum of most staff training programs for dementia care. Although a minimum of 8 hours of dementia care training is recommended for staff who provide direct care, the amount of time devoted to behavior management varies and is limited usually to one or two classroom sessions. It is essential that the sequence of topics in training programs be consistent so that each class builds on the knowledge learned in the previous one. All training programs in dementia care should include the following topics:

1. An understanding of the different types of dementia and behaviors that are characteristic of those dementias; descriptions of the progression of cognitive impairment and its effect on feelings and behavior
2. The application of communication skills in behavior management strategies such as the use of eye contact; touch; verbal and nonverbal cues; and short, simple sentences
3. The use of environmental modifications to prevent and manage problem behaviors, including the reduction of noise and activity; the provision of safe, secured wandering areas; and creation of a homelike atmosphere

4. The use of strategies that help to build a supportive relationship between the staff and residents and help to meet the psychosocial needs of the residents; staff approaches such as validation, reminiscence, and the encouragement of personal choice should be taught
5. An understanding of the use of chemical and physical restraints in managing problem behaviors, their effects on people with dementia, and the need to develop alternative interventions
6. The use of behavior-specific documentation to chart and track behavior disorders
7. The creation of a partnership with residents' family members in order to develop and implement care plans for managing problem behaviors
8. Methods for reducing and handling the stress associated with caring for people with dementia

TRAINING PROGRAMS

Many good staff training programs for dementia care are available. Table 1 lists several models that emphasize training in behavior management. Additional training programs and resources are provided in the appendix at the end of the chapter.

TRAINERS

People who provide training in dementia care come from diverse educational and professional backgrounds. The responsibility for staff education in long-term care settings is often assigned to the director of staff development/education, who is usually a nurse with an R.N. or B.S.N. degree. This individual may be capable of training staff in the areas of basic patient care and infection control and quality control issues, but may not have the expertise needed to conduct training in dementia care. Therapeutic ways of handling the behaviors associated with dementia should be taught by someone who has extensive knowledge of dementing illness and related psychodynamics, as well as an understanding of basic psychopathology and clinical interventions, such as a psychiatric nurse, a licensed clinical social worker, or a psychologist. In addition to possessing the necessary clinical credentials, a trainer in behavior management must have experience not only in working with people with dementia but in teaching all levels of staff. For programs without such a qualified person on staff, it may be necessary to contract with a professional from the community to provide at least the behavioral segment of dementia care training. This person can provide train-the-trainer education to designated staff in order to encourage continuing education and follow-up training. Many Alzheimer's Association chapters provide assistance with staff training in dementia care and provide training materials.

Table 1. Behavior management training programs

Program	Description	Target audience
Aggressive Behavior Education Program (Feldt & Ryden, 1992)	Prior to training, a dementia-knowledge pretest is administered along with 2 additional instruments (characteristics of residents and experience of caregiving) Instruction in cognitive losses, precipitants of aggression, communication techniques, strategies for preventing aggressive behavior, and managing personal feelings Use of role modeling direct care of residents develops skills in working with residents with cognitive impairment who are aggressive	Nursing assistants in long-term care settings
Calming Aggressive Reactions in the Elderly Program (Mentes & Ferrario, 1989)	Identification of risk factors in aggression Use of preventive approaches Demonstrates calming techniques Use of protective intervention when other approaches do not work	Nursing assistants in nursing facilities
FOCUSED (Ripich, 1994; Ripich, Wykle, & Niles, 1995)	Consists of 6 2-hour modules that focus on 7 communication strategies • AD and associated communication and language decline • Differences among normal forgetting, depression, and AD • Value of interpersonal skills in care of residents with AD • Cultural and ethical issues involved in communicating with residents with AD • Stages of AD and concurrent communication characteristics • Use and evaluation of FOCUSED strategies and techniques for promoting effective communication between caregivers and family members with AD	Nursing assistants who care for people with Alzheimer's disease (AD)
GENTLECARE (Jones & Wright, 1991)	Understanding pathology and implications of progressive dementing illness Increase staff awareness of residents' ecology, relationships, and the context in which they live	Multidisciplinary staff in dementia-specific residential care settings and geropsychiatric units

(continued)

51

Table 1—continued

Program	Description	Target audience
GENTLECARE—continued	Staff engages in creative problem solving with goal of allowing residents to function at their highest level possible	Nursing staff
Management of Catastrophic Reactions in Dementia Victims (Williams, 1994)	Empathy training, using VCR and monitor, tape player with headphones, and strobe light to overstimulate participants and help them "step into another's shoes"	
	Theory training, involving instruction in functioning of demented and nondemented brains	
	Skills training to assist staff in creating stimulation-reducing environments and familiar daily routines for residents	
R.E.S.P.E.C.T. (Maxfield, Lewis, & Cannon, 1996)	Examine staff approaches used in assisting residents	Nursing staff (NA, LPNs, and RNs) in geropsychiatric hospitals
	Introduce methods of recognize, empathize, support, prevent, enhance, care, and take time	
	Demonstrate and have staff practice methods	
	Follow-up with observation, consultation, and support to staff on units	

It is essential that any training component that addresses the personal feelings of staff about their jobs and the stress of caring for people with dementia not be conducted by supervisors or other management staff. This particular segment of dementia training should be provided in a nonthreatening environment in which staff feel comfortable discussing the anger and frustration that they may experience in caring for residents with dementia.

TRAINING METHODS

It has been suggested that providing classroom instruction in the management of behavior disorders in dementia care is ineffective without the inclusion of other teaching methods (Orr-Rainey, 1991), such as videotapes, case examples, and role plays. Videotapes serve as an effective orientation to older adults with dementia by providing a visual overview of the disease as portrayed by real-life people with dementia and their families. Videotapes are also excellent tools for demonstrating situations involving problem behaviors and staff approaches, as well as for stimulating discussion.

Case examples are effective teaching tools in addressing behavior disorders. Situations taken from resident charts as well as examples of past and current cases contributed by staff can be used for group discussion. Strategies for addressing these situations can then be discussed and can include examining possible precipitating factors leading to the behavior as well as ways in which the behavior could have been prevented.

Role playing can be a useful learning activity in demonstrating methods in which to apply new knowledge and skills. Typical situations involving resident behavior disorders are enacted, with staff playing the roles of residents, staff, and, in some cases, family members. These exercises provide staff with the opportunity to practice newly learned skills while allowing for input and discussion from the rest of the class. Special attention should be paid to situations (e.g., bathing, toileting, eating) in which problem behaviors frequently occur. Role-playing these and other situations involving problem behaviors not only provides the opportunity to reenact behaviors and responses but also promotes the development of strategies to reduce the occurrence of future incidents.

MEASUREMENT TOOLS

Pre- and posttests are important tools for use in measuring changes in knowledge and attitude; the pretest also can be employed as a teaching tool. Reviewing the questions and answers with the class following the administration of the test allows for further discussion of the subject matter and identifies gaps in knowledge that can help trainers plan subsequent training sessions. Often, posttests that assess an increase in knowledge are administered immediately following the training series. Additional posttests administered several months after training may provide some indication of the long-term effects of training.

In addition to written tests, an increase in knowledge and skills can be assessed by random observations of staff interactions with residents with dementia. Examples of observations that can be documented and rated include the following:

- Providing choices to residents when appropriate
- Validating residents' realities and concerns
- Responding to persistent residents in a calm, patient manner
- Instructing residents in a basic step-by-step process
- Encouraging residents' attempts to maintain remaining capabilities
- Using behavior management strategies, such as redirection and defusion, taught in training sessions

Another measurable indicator of training effectiveness is a reduction in the number of incidents involving problem behaviors. This reduction is best achieved through the use of special charting for behaviors and assessment instruments that are designed to identify problem behaviors. Many of these tools can be used to measure the occurrence of specific behaviors and provide quantitative data with which to gauge the effectiveness of staff training. The Disruptive Behavior Rating Scale (Mungas, Weiler, Franzi, & Henry, 1989) can be used to communicate resident behaviors to staff and requires a minimal amount of time to complete. The Brief Behavioral Symptom Rating Scale is another instrument designed to focus on observable behavior and can be filled out by individuals who have no formal psychiatric training (Rabins, 1994). The Behavior Monitoring Chart (Rader & Harvath, 1991) measures resident behaviors every 2 hours during a 24-hour period and can be adjusted to measure the occurrence and severity of the behaviors.

The use of visual graphs to document behaviors helps to identify patterns as well as antecedents to the behavior and consequences from interventions. One such graph is the Behavior Flow Sheet (McAliley, Ashenberg, & Maier, 1996), which can include information on the target behavior, the date and time that it occurred, the setting in which it took place, the people who were present, and the intervention that was used. The Behavior Flow Sheet can be designed in such a way as to provide the data collector with a picture of the behavior pattern.

In order for training effectiveness to be measured accurately, the target behaviors should be identified and baseline data collected prior to staff training. Comparisons or baseline data and the data collected following the training program provide a feedback mechanism for assessing changes in the number of situations involving the target behaviors as well as changes in the types of staff interventions used. Flow sheets not only serve as a mechanism for evaluating training effectiveness but provide a direction for care planning as well.

ONGOING TRAINING

Staff training in dementia behavior management must extend beyond the classroom-style experience of knowledge and skill building. Training should include the use of interactive problem solving, taking advantage of "teachable moments" following training, and periodic in-service training sessions. "Teachable moments" are actual situations occurring in a dementia care program that provide the opportunity for staff to apply the behavior management techniques learned in the classroom setting. This follow-up instruction requires staff trainers to spend time in the dementia program in an unobtrusive manner in order to observe staff intervention in difficult situations. It should be remembered that the trainer's role in this situation is as an observer and, in most cases, should not interfere with the staff's attempt to handle the residents' behavior. The time to evaluate the staff's actions should come immediately following the incident, with the trainer providing either positive feedback or constructive criticism, as well as suggestions for future incidents. Under no circumstances should staff be reprimanded for inappropriate handling of a difficult situation in the presence of other staff, residents, or residents' family members. Immediate intervention by a trainer or other staff should take place only when the resident or staff is at risk for harm. If the trainer is constantly intervening in situations involving difficult behaviors, the staff may continue to seek assistance from the trainer when confronted with a problem instead of attempting to apply the behavior management techniques learned in dementia training. The following case example demonstrates the successful application of classroom learning to practice and the impact of that experience on the staff member.

> Deanna, a nursing assistant, had recently completed a series of training sessions on dementia care, but she was not totally "sold" on the approaches to behavior management that were taught in the classes. The one strategy that she was having particular difficulty accepting was the instructor's recommendation to validate the residents' concerns and to "go along with their reality," regardless of whether it was accurate. "I'd feel foolish pretending to go along with residents' statements that weren't true," she argued, "and besides, it's wrong to lie to them." Several weeks later, Deanna found herself having to persuade Mrs. Bartolowsky to go to the dining room for her meal. Becoming increasingly agitated, Mrs. Bartolowsky refused to leave her room because she insisted that there were children playing under her bed. After several unsuccessful attempts at reality orientation, Deanna decided to use the approach taught in dementia care training. After looking around to see if anyone was watching her, she knelt down by Mrs. Bartolowsky's bed and chased the children away. After reassuring Mrs. Bartolowsky that the children were gone, Deanna escorted her to the dining room. A few

days later, she sought out the training instructor to tell her that she had been successful in managing the situation and that this feeling of success had changed her opinion of this approach to behavior management.

In addition to providing dementia training to new staff, administration should offer regular in-services that specifically address behavior management. In the 11 years that the author has provided dementia training to staff in hospitals, nursing facilities, assisted living facilities, adult day programs, and home health care, behavior management continues to be the topic that staff requests most often.

CONCLUSION

Behaviors associated with dementia need to be considered from the perspective of the older adult with cognitive impairment. Such consideration allows staff to attempt to determine the reason for the behavior. No magic formulas consistently resolve the problems encountered by staff who care for older people with dementia, but providing them with a variety of approaches and strategies that promote confidence and competence will improve staff morale, decrease turnover, and, most important, improve the quality of dementia care.

REFERENCES

Austrom, M. (1996). Training staff to work in special care. In S.B. Hoffman & M. Kaplan (Eds.), *Special care programs for people with dementia* (pp. 17–35). Baltimore: Health Professions Press.

Bridges-Parlet, S., Knopman, D., & Thompson, T. (1994). Descriptive study of physically aggressive behavior in dementia by direct observation. *Journal of the American Geriatrics Society, 42*, 192–197.

Dougherty, L., Bolger, J., Preston, D., Jones, S., & Payne, H. (1992). Effects of exposure to aggressive behavior on job satisfaction of health care staff. *Journal of Applied Gerontology, 11*, 160–172.

Feldt, K.S., & Ryden, M.B. (1992). Aggressive behavior: Educating nursing assistants. *Journal of Gerontological Nursing, 18*(5), 3–12.

Gerdner, L.A., & Buckwalter, K.C. (1996). Review of state policies regarding special care units: Implications for family consumers and health care professionals. *American Journal of Alzheimer's Disease, H*(2), 16–27.

Henderson, J.N. (1987). Dementia-specific care units in nursing homes. What's so special? Do they work? In J.N. Henderson & E. Pfeiffer (Eds.), *The family caregiver: Lifeline to the frail patient* (pp. 122–130). Tampa: University of South Florida Suncoast Gerontology Center.

Jayaratne, S., & Chess, W. (1986). Job stress, job deficit, emotional support, and competence: Their relationship to burnout. *Journal of Applied Social Sciences, 10*, 135–155.

Jones, M., & Wright, J. (1991). *Beyond love: A resource book for caregiver support and education*. Burnaby, B.C., Canada: Moyra Jones Resources.

Kaplan, M. (1996a). Challenges to success. In S.B. Hoffman & M. Kaplan (Eds.), *Special care programs for people with dementia* (pp. 1–15). Baltimore: Health Professions Press.

Kaplan, M. (1996b). *Clinical practice with caregivers of dementia patients.* Washington, DC: Taylor & Francis.

Leiter, M.P., & Maslach, C. (1988). The impact of interpersonal environment on burnout and organizational commitment. *Journal of Organizational Behavior, 9,* 297–308.

Maxfield, M.C., Lewis, R.E., & Cannon, S. (1996). Training staff to prevent aggressive behavior of cognitively impaired elderly patients during bathing and grooming. *Journal of Gerontological Nursing, 22*(1), 37–43.

McAliley, L.G., Ashenberg, M.D., & Maier, N.L. (1996). The behavioral flow sheet. *Nurse Practitioner, 21*(6), 22–40.

Mentes, J., & Ferrario, J. (1989). Calming aggressive reactions: A preventive program. *Journal of Gerontological Nursing, 15*(2), 22–27.

Mobily, P., Maas, M., Buckwalter, K.C., & Kelly, L. (1992). Staff stress on an Alzheimer's unit. *Journal of Psychosocial Nursing, 30*(9), 25–31.

Mungas, D., Weiler, P., Franzi, C., & Henry, R. (1989). Assessment of disruptive behavior associated with dementia: The Disruptive Behavior Rating Scales. *Journal of Geriatric Psychiatry and Neurology, 2*(4), 196–202.

Novak, M., & Chappell, N.L. (1994). Nursing assistant burnout and the cognitively impaired elderly. *International Journal of Aging & Human Development, 39*(2), 105–120.

Orr-Rainey, N.K. (1991). Establishing a dementia unit. In P.D. Sloane & L.J. Mathew (Eds.), *Dementia units in long-term care* (pp. 5b–5o). Baltimore: The Johns Hopkins University Press.

Peppard, N.R. (1986). Special nursing home units for residents with primary degenerative dementia: Alzheimer's disease. *Journal of Gerontological Social Work, 9,* 5–13.

Rabins, P.V. (1994). The validity of a caregiver-rated brief behavior symptom rating scale (BSRS) for use in the cognitively impaired. *International Journal of Geriatric Psychiatry, 9,* 205–210.

Rader, J., & Harvath, T. (1991). How to document difficult behavior. *Geriatric Nursing, 12* (5), 231–232.

Ripich, D.N. (1994). Functional communication with AD patients: A caregiver training program. *Alzheimer Disease and Associated Disorders, An International Journal, 8*(Suppl. 3), 95–109.

Ripich, D.N., Wykle, M., & Niles, S. (1995). Alzheimer's disease caregivers: The FOCUSED Program. *Gerontological Nursing, 16*(1), 15–19.

Vance, A., & Davidhizar, D. (1997). Motivating the paraprofessional in long-term care. *Health Care Supervisor, 15*(4), 57–64.

Williams, J.K. (1994). Evolution of a specialty unit in response to a changing patient population: Providing workers with specific information and getting them involved in creating change is the best way to lift spirits and turn a crisis around. *Geriatric Nursing, 15*(3), 151–153.

APPENDIX
TRAINING RESOURCES[1]

Training Programs

Alzheimer's 101: The Basics for Caregiving
Columbia, SC: South Carolina Education Television Network, 1989
Phone (800) 553-7752

Videotape, trainer's manual, and a learner's guide that address the various aspects of Alzheimer's disease and care, including communication, behavior, personal care, activities, and caregiver stress.
Price: Video: $305.00 (purchase), $160.00 (rental); trainer's manual: $12.00 (quantity discount); learner's guide: $9.95 (quantity discount)

Caring for People with Alzheimer's Disease: A Training Manual for Direct Care Providers
Gayle Andresen, R.N.-C., M.S., A.N.P./G.N.P., in association with Health Education Development System, Inc., and Cooperative Health Education Program
Baltimore: Health Professions Press, 1995
Phone (888) 337-8808

Provides a complete curriculum for training staff in dementia care. Topics covered include communication techniques, managing difficult behaviors, and personal care. Sample quizzes and handouts are provided.
Price: $26.95

Creative Interventions with the Alzheimer's Patient
Radium Springs, NM: Geriatric Resources Inc., 1992
Phone (505) 524-0250

Three videotapes and a training manual that discuss behaviors exhibited by people with Alzheimer's disease, functional assessment tools, and interventions.
Price: Complete set: $345.00; tapes 1 and 2 only: $255.00; tape 3 only: $134.00

For Those Who Take Care: An Alzheimer's Disease Training Program for Nursing Assistants
B.J. Helm and D.R. Wekstein
Lexington: University of Kentucky Alzheimer's Disease Center, 1991; available from the Alzheimer's Disease Education and Referral Center (ADEAR)
Phone (800) 438-4380

A training manual and 45 slides that include information about Alzheimer's disease, caregiving issues, and behavior management.
Price: $55.00

---

[1]Prices are subject to change and were accurate to the best of the author's and publisher's knowledge at the time of publication.

Keys to Better Care: A Training Program for Nursing Home Staff Caring for People with Alzheimer's Disease and Related Dementia

Narbeth, PA: Consult Services, Inc., 1991
Phone (800) 653-0480

Seven videotapes and a two-volume trainer's manual are designed to provide assistance in planning dementia care programs and training staff in dementia care. Several modules focus on problem behaviors. Also included in the training package is a seven-volume reference library and a 1-year subscription to the *American Journal of Alzheimer's Care and Related Disorders and Research*.
Price: $2,500.00 (quantity discounts available)

Managing and Understanding Behavior Problems in Alzheimer's Disease and Related Disorders

Linda Teri, Ph.D.
Baltimore: Health Professions Press
Phone (888) 337-8808

A series of 10 videotapes accompanied by a training manual that address specific behavior problems related to dementia.
Price: $295.00

Nurses' Aides—Making a Difference: Skills for Managing Difficult Behaviors in Dementia Victims

Dallas: University of Texas Southwestern Medical Center, 1991; available from the Alzheimer's Disease Education and Referral Center (ADEAR)
Phone (800) 438-4380

A 30-minute videotape and viewing guide that demonstrate appropriate interventions in managing problem behaviors.
Price: $20.00

Speaking for Them: Identifying Psychiatric Complications in Alzheimer's Patients

San Diego: Alzheimer's Disease Center, University of California, San Diego, 1991; available from the Alzheimer's Disease Education and Referral Center (ADEAR)
Phone (800) 438-4380

A 13-minute videotape that identifies psychiatric complications of Alzheimer's disease. A manual is included that describes behavioral aspects of Alzheimer's disease and their management.
Price: $18.00

Videos

Behaviors Associated with Dementia: Case Presentations

Baltimore: University of Maryland School of Medicine
Phone (800) 328-7450

Documents actual experiences of residents of nursing facilities who exhibit behaviors associated with dementia, providing a stimulus for class discussion.
Price: $300.00 (purchase), $100.00 (rental)

Caring for Disordered Behavior in the Nursing Home
Baltimore: University of Maryland School of Medicine
Phone (800) 328-7450

Documented episodes of problem behaviors in residents of nursing facilities and interviews with staff identifying appropriate interventions.
Price: $300.00 (purchase), $100.00 (rental)

Dress Him While He Walks: Behavior Management in Caring for Residents with Alzheimer's Disease
Global Village Communications
Available through Terra Nova Films
Phone (800) 779-8491

Demonstrates how to identify the causes of problem behaviors and how to use creative approaches to develop an individual behavior management plan for each person with dementia.
Price: $145.00

Managing the Resident with Dementia: Specific Nursing Strategies
Baltimore: University of Maryland School of Medicine
Phone (800) 328-7450

Documents actual resident behaviors and provides management strategies.
Price: $300.00 (purchase), $100.00 (rental)

Nurse's Aides: Making a Difference
Chicago: Terra Nova Films
Phone (800) 779-8491

Introduces basic concepts for handling difficult behaviors of residents with dementia, using vignettes of residents demonstrating the behaviors and staff experimenting with different interventions.
Price: $95.00 (purchase), $40.00 (rental)

The Nursing Home Mental Health Series
Baltimore: University of Maryland School of Medicine
Phone (800) 328-7450

Reviews the most common behavior problems that occur in the nursing facility and outlines practical approaches to minimize their occurrence and strategies to manage them effectively.
Price: $1,000.00 (series of 7 videos); $200 (individual videos for purchase), $100.00 (individual videos for rental)

Solving Bathing Problems in Persons with Alzheimer's Disease and Related Dementias

Philip D. Sloane, M.D., M.P.H., Ann Louise Barrick, Ph.D., and Vanessa Honn
Baltimore: Health Professions Press
(888) 337-8808

A videotape accompanied by an instruction book that teaches staff to understand problem behaviors that occur during bathing and to utilize strategies to make bathing easier for residents with dementia and staff.
Price: $129.00 (purchase)

Books

Care of Alzheimer's Patients: A Manual for Nursing Home Staff
Lisa P. Gwyther, M.S.W.
Chicago: Alzheimer's Disease and Related Disorders Association, Inc., and American Health Care Association, 1985

Comforting the Confused: Strategies for Managing Dementia
Stephanie B. Hoffman, Ph.D., and Connie Platt, M.A.
New York: Springer Publishing, 1991

Special Care Programs for People with Dementia
Stephanie B. Hoffman, Ph.D., and Mary Kaplan, M.S.W., L.C.S.W., A.C.S.W.
Baltimore: Health Professions Press, 1996

Additional Resources

Alzheimer's Association materials
Chicago: Alzheimer's Association
Phone (800) 272-3900

A catalog of videos, booklets, fact sheets, manuals, and kits on Alzheimer's disease and related disorders.

Caring and Sharing: A Catalog of Training Materials from Alzheimer's Disease Centers
Silver Spring, MD: Alzheimer's Disease Education and Referral Center (ADEAR)
Phone (800) 438-4380

5

Nurturing

Stephanie B. Hoffman, Ph.D.

Every human being requires nurturing, from the youngest premature infant to the oldest adult with cognitive impairment. Interventions to improve dementia care have included environmental modifications, medications, and behavior management training programs (e.g., see Hiatt, 1989; Smith, Buckwalter, & Mitchell, 1993). Nancy Mace's (1993) observations of international dementia programs suggest that people with dementia are responsive to subtle changes in their environment. The programs with the best outcomes, based on her naturalistic observations of individuals' behavior, seem to emphasize a caring approach by staff.

It has been suggested that the ability to nurture is a key aspect of providing high-quality care to older adults with dementia. Research by Hoffman, Platt, Hamill, and Barry (1986) indicates that such individuals are still very much affected by nonverbal communication, such as touch and tone of voice. This aspect of nurturing is important. Tender, loving care may be the most effective intervention for improving the quality of life of individuals with dementia. Providing care in this manner also may enhance the morale and enjoyment of caregivers.

According to Clarke and Hornick (1984) and Erikson (1950), nurturance is the affectional component of interaction. A more general definition is to promote development by providing nourishment, support, encouragement, and other physical and emotional supports during the stages of growth. Being nurtured is of primary importance in the development of self-acceptance based on a feeling of being loved. The primary relationship for providing and receiving nurturing is the parent–child dyad, but all humans have a need for nurturing throughout life. Good friends also provide love, affection, and encouragement. Bell and Troxel (1997) suggest that caregivers should relate to people with dementia as they would a best friend.

NURTURING AND THE HIERARCHY OF NEEDS

As people with dementia regress, nurturing needs increase, ultimately matching those of children. As the cortex deteriorates, the most basic human needs take precedence. The author suggests that these needs reflect those in Maslow's (1968) hierarchy of needs. Higher-level needs take precedence at earlier stages of dementia; lower-level needs become most important at advanced stages. At the top of the needs hierarchy is self-actualization. People at this stage are creative and open to new experiences. This level of needs is immediately affected by dementia; people tend to decompensate (i.e., loss of physiological compensation or psychological balance) in new environments and cope with anxiety using tried-and-true coping methods. Nurturing at this stage means that caregivers accept the shrinking world of loved ones and help to decrease their anxiety by taking over stressful responsibilities.

Self-esteem needs are at the next-lower rung of the hierarchy. At this level, individuals want respect. People with dementia may hide memory loss and confabulate forgotten incidents. However, caregivers should not confront them about untruths but should instead validate them. At this needs stage, older adults with dementia may also abandon activities that they can no longer perform to former personal standards. A nurturing caregiver respects that people with dementia may need to relinquish formerly satisfying hobbies and instead engage in less complex activities. Teri and Logsdon (1991) developed a list of potentially satisfying activities for people with dementia. These activities are simple—being outside, listening to music, laughing, being complimented, being told they are loved, and discussing past events. The activities should not exceed their capacity for performing them because frustration rather than enjoyment may be the outcome. Teri and Logsdon believe that consistent engagement in pleasant activities may relieve the depression that is common among people with cognitive impairment.

Attachment is the next level of need in Maslow's hierarchy. This need is that of loving and being loved, of belonging. People with cognitive impairment find it difficult to reciprocate love. Although they may feel gratitude for the care being provided, they may have trouble expressing thanks. The nurturing caregiver must show dramatically that he or she cares. Nurturing this need means demonstrating love through smiles, warm hugs, and much patience. Without sufficient nurturing, people with dementia begin to disengage, to withdraw, from the environment. Wandering may increase as people with cognitive impairment look for love and former attachments. They may feel that they do not belong to this new environment; they feel lost in it. Even at home, they may fail to recognize their spouse or loved ones. Nurturing caregivers should not feel hurt when they are not recognized; they should provide care graciously and repeat their name frequently to the person with dementia.

Satisfaction of attachment needs also suggests that individuals with dementia must be allowed to nurture others. Camp et al. (1997) asked people with mild to moderate cognitive impairment to teach children using Montessori methods. The participants conducted these intergenerational sessions once a week for 30–45 minutes. Camp and colleagues found many positive benefits to their program: Older residents of a dementia-specific care unit (DSCU) or adult day setting could indeed serve as mentors to young children, disengagement was prevented, and participants felt proud of their remaining abilities.

As the cognitive capabilities of people with dementia regress, the next need on the hierarchy that must be satisfied is that of safety. Safety needs include security and comfort. People with cognitive impairment should live in a secure environment. This environment should be safe and predictable, yet homelike. Although the setting may be locked, it should never feel like a prison to the residents. Alarms should not go off constantly. Adequate programming that is geared to a level that satisfies residents should be scheduled. An adequate number of nursing and activities staff should be in place. The environment should include homelike possessions, pictures, and objects to manipulate and enjoy. Residents should be free of pain and comfortable.

The lowest-level need on Maslow's hierarchy is that of biological needs. As older adults reach an advanced stage of dementia, biological needs take precedence. Personal needs focus on activities of daily living (ADLs)—feeding, toileting, and touching. Nurturing caregivers feed residents with advanced dementia slowly and patiently. Foods that residents remember from childhood (e.g., ice cream, milkshakes, oatmeal, Jell-O, mashed potatoes) may be the most comforting to them. Nurturing caregivers do not rush feeding; it may take 30–60 minutes to thoroughly feed an individual with advanced dementia. People with this level of cognitive impairment also should be massaged, cuddled, and sung to. At this lowest need level, people's needs are similar to those of babies. Babies love hugs, cuddles, play, naps, simple songs—activities that are also enjoyed by older adults with dementia.

NURTURING AND POSITIVE INFANTILIZATION

The word *infantilization* implies treating people as if they were infants, a derogatory or negative meaning. However, the infantilization of people with dementia is not disrespectful. It is actually respectful of the emotional and physical needs of the person. If a person with dementia benefits from a singsong tone of voice, a gentle hug, a doll to cuddle, comfort foods, or pleasant music or lullabies, these interventions should be provided. If the person prefers to be called "Baby" or "Papa," such names are not disrespectful. The author has observed that residents of DSCUs brighten up and appear more oriented when addressed by their nicknames or by other "sweet" names.

Some staff members may react against treating people with dementia as though they were toddlers or infants. However, given the severe regression of such individuals, this sort of treatment may be what they need in order to thrive. The affect and neediness of people with dementia elicits from staff and loved ones a "caretaker" or "motherese" pattern of speech and behavior. This instinctual response promotes both the survival of infants and the survival of the neediest older adults.

NURTURING IN THE PREVENTION OF ABUSE

A program to enhance nurturing by caregivers of people with dementia may decrease their own stress, increase their morale and use of nurturing techniques, and, ultimately, lower the amount of abuse leveled against people with dementia. As a result of such a program people with dementia will display fewer agitated behaviors (e.g., resistance to care, wandering, combativeness) and feel increased comfort and morale. An empathy training workshop designed by Williams, Wood, and Moorleghen (1994) had this very effect. Staff on a DSCU were trained to empathize with residents with dementia who were overstimulated. The training staff asked a volunteer to experience concomitant multiple stimuli—a radio, a strobe light, a memorization task to a video, a serial sevens' task, and an ADL task (putting on a sweater while conversing with a staff member). The volunteer and audience felt the severe confusion caused by overstimulation. Residents' records of combative behavior showed a significant lessening of incidents following staff training in empathy and other nurturing skills.

The long-term consequences of nurturing such as reduced abuse of older adults must be studied. Nurturing interventions in the parenting field show that abuse decreases as caregiver nurturing skills increase (Bavolek, 1990). Although not reported frequently, abuse (e.g., physical, verbal, sexual, financial) of older adults with dementia by their caregivers is high. Often, abuse is the result of the stress of providing care to people who are challenging to work with (Bowie & Mountain, 1993; Coyne, 1991; Haley & Coleton, 1992; Holt, 1993; Vinton, 1992).

The selection of appropriate staff for a DSCU is critically important. Staff who have a desire to work in a DSCU and who are open to training should be selected. Their prior work experience and their potential criminal background must be reviewed carefully. During the employment interview, questions as to how the interviewee handled his or her most difficult client or resident in the past can be addressed. The interviewer should assess the candidate's level of empathy and compassion and nonverbal communication abilities (e.g., La Monica, 1986).

The qualities of a good preschool teacher—patience, a sympathetic approach, ability to communicate with the person on his or her level, a gentle touch, tolerance for easily expressed emotion, and empathy with frustration—are the qualities that should be sought in a nurturing caregiver.

ENHANCED NURTURING

A variety of types of literature contribute background information to the concept of enhanced nurturing. These include empathy training programs, parenting training programs, abuse literature, hospice literature, existing training programs for caregivers of people with dementia, and literature on nonverbal communication (e.g., touch).

From the classical literature on professional touch, it is noted that older people with dementia are the least physically touched of any age group by nursing personnel (Barnett, 1972). Typically, nursing staff use procedural rather than comfort touching as part of their daily care routine. Also, nursing staff converse only minimally with people with dementia (Blondis & Jackson, 1982). Although this lack of contact can be attributed to time limitations, it may also be the result of lack of training in how to properly interact with older adults with cognitive impairment. A study by Hoffman, Platt, and Barry (1987) found that nursing staff used inappropriate interventions when trying to manage their most difficult resident and consequently felt frustrated, depressed, and helpless. According to Heiselman and Noelker (1991), nursing assistants believe themselves to be nurturing and compassionate. However, half of the residents in the study complained that nursing assistants were neither sensitive nor responsive to residents' feelings.

NURTURING TRAINING PROGRAMS

Hoffman and associates (1986–1988) conducted a series of studies that examined nonverbal communication, confirming that nonverbal communication abilities are preserved even in people with profound cognitive impairment. A training manual, *Comforting the Confused: Strategies for Managing Dementia* (Hoffman & Platt, 1991), highlights nonverbal communication as a critical intervention for providing comfort to people with dementia. Evaluation research on several chapters in the book showed that nurses increased their knowledge, felt more competent, and reported using more nonverbal techniques after training.

The Calming Aggressive Reactions in the Elderly (C.A.R.E.) training program (Mentes & Ferrario, 1989) taught nursing assistants to prevent resident aggression through the use of verbal and nonverbal communication, touch, and facilitation of a therapeutic relationship. Following the program, fewer incidents of resident abuse of staff occurred.

The approach to training staff of a DSCU should emphasize the contrast between regular care and nurturing care. In an enhanced nurturing program, various elements of communication should be highlighted and practiced. The use of praise and encouragement should be emphasized. Simple statements should be used and should be articulated slowly, with a 5-second pause to wait for the person with dementia to respond. Soothing touch should be carefully taught. A lilting tone of voice must be used in appropriate settings. Songs and a sense of humor are recommended, and patience and kindness must be demonstrated.

EVALUATION APPROACHES

Evaluation measures to test the effectiveness of an enhanced nurturing training program would include several of the following: a caregiver version of the Nurturance Inventory (Clarke & Hornick, 1984), staff empathy skills, use of positive nonverbal communication skills, caregiver burden, caregiver morale, and inclusion of nurturing interventions in resident care plans.

The behavior of people with dementia should be monitored regularly using the Minimum Data Set. The level of discomfort should be observed by the Discomfort Scale (Hurley, Volicer, Hanrahan, Houde, & Volicer, 1992), which is an objective scale for measuring discomfort in noncommunicative people with Alzheimer's disease. The frequency of problem behaviors can be assessed via a variety of observational measures (Cohen-Mansfield, Marx, & Rosenthal, 1989). Resident depression should be assessed by mental health professionals.

CONCLUSION

An enhanced nurturing program can be adapted to the needs of any target group. Often, professional caregivers feel compassion stress and compassion fatigue (Figley, 1995), and they feel additionally stressed by family complaints and negativity (Heiselman & Noelker, 1991). These caregivers need a great deal of support. Families can participate in an enhanced nurturing training program and use the skills they have learned with both their family members and facility staff. If staff received more nurturing from families and if families and people with dementia received nurturing from staff, the emotional climate of DSCUs would be positive indeed.

REFERENCES

Barnett, K. (1972). A survey of the current utilization of touch by health team personnel with hospitalized patients. *International Journal of Nursing Studies, 9,* 195–209.
Bavolek, S.J. (1990). *Research and validation report of the nurturing programs: Effective family-based approaches to treating and preventing child abuse and neglect.* Park City, UT: Family Development Resources, Inc.

Bell, V., & Troxel, D. (1997). *The best friends approach to Alzheimer's care.* Baltimore: Health Professions Press.

Blondis, M.N., & Jackson, B.E. (1982). *Nonverbal communication with patients: Back to the human touch* (2nd ed.). New York: John Wiley & Sons.

Bowie, P., & Mountain, G. (1993). Life on a long stay ward: Extracts from the diary of an observing researcher. *International Journal of Geriatric Psychiatry, 8*(12), 1001–1007.

Camp, C.J., Judge, K.S., Bye, C.A., Fox, K.M., Bowden, J., Bell, M., Valencic, K., & Mattern, J.M. (1997). An intergenerational program for persons with dementia using Montessori methods. *Gerontologist, 37*(5), 688–692.

Clarke, M., & Hornick, J. (1984). The development of the Nurturance Inventory: An instrument for assessing parenting practices. *Child Psychiatry and Human Development, 14*(1), 49–63.

Cohen-Mansfield, J., Marx, M.S., & Rosenthal, A.S. (1989). A description of agitation in nursing home residents. *Journal of Gerontology: Medical Sciences, 36*(3),150–158.

Coyne, A.C. (1991). Relationship between cognitive impairment and elder abuse. In T. Tatara, & M.M Rittman (Eds.), *Findings of five elder abuse studies from the NARCEA research grants program* (pp. 3–20). Washington, DC: NARCEA.

Erikson, E.H. (1950). *Childhood and society.* New York: W.W. Norton.

Figley, C.R. (1995). Compassion fatigue: Toward a new understanding of the costs of caring. In B. Judnall Stamm (Ed.), *Secondary traumatic stress: Self-care issues for clinicians, researchers, and educators* (pp. 3–28). Lutherville, MD: Sidran Press.

Haley, W.E., & Coleton, M.I. (1992). Alzheimer's disease: Special issues in elder abuse and neglect. *Journal of Elder Abuse and Neglect, 4*(4), 71–85.

Heiselman, T., & Noelker, L.S. (1991). Enhancing mutual respect among nursing assistants, residents, and residents' families. *Gerontologist, 31*(4), 552–555.

Hiatt, L.G. (1989). Design and mentally impaired persons: Considerations of the sophisticated sponsor. In H.J. Altman & B.N. Altman (Eds.), *Alzheimer's and Parkinson's diseases.* New York: Plenum Press.

Hoffman, S.B. (1988). The importance of nonverbal communication in the care of people with Alzheimer's disease. *American Journal of Alzheimer's Care and Research, 3*(1), 25–30.

Hoffman, S.B., & Platt, C.A. (1991). *Comforting the confused: Strategies for managing dementia.* New York: Springer Publishing.

Hoffman, S.B., Platt, C.A., & Barry, K.E. (1987). Managing the difficult nursing home patient: The impact on untrained nursing home staff. *American Journal of Alzheimer's Care and Research, 2*(4), 26–31.

Hoffman, S.B., Platt, C.A., Hamill, L.A., & Barry, K.E. (1986). When language fails: Nonverbal communication abilities of the demented. In A.D. Kenny & J.T. Hutton (Eds.), *Senile dementia of the Alzheimer's type.* New York: Alan R. Liss.

Holt, M.G. (1993). Elder sexual abuse in Britain: Preliminary findings. *Journal of Elder Abuse and Neglect, 5*(2), 63–71.

Hurley, A.C., Volicer, B.J., Hanrahan, P.A., Houde, S., & Volicer, L. (1992). Assessment of discomfort in advanced Alzheimer patients. *Research in Nursing and Health, 15*(5), 369–377.

La Monica, E.L. (1986). *La Monica empathy profile.* Tuxedo, NY: XICOM.

Mace, N.L. (1993, May/June). Observations of dementia specific care around the world. *American Journal of Alzheimer's Care and Related Disorders & Research,* pp. 1–8.

Maslow, A. (1968). *Toward a psychology of being*. Princeton, NJ: Van Nostrand Reinhold.

Mentes, J.C., & Ferrario, J. (1989). Calming aggressive reactions: A preventive program. *Journal of Gerontological Nursing, 15*(2), 22–27.

Smith, M., Buckwalter, K., & Mitchell, S. (1993). *Geriatric mental health training series*. New York: Springer Publishing.

Teri, L., & Logsdon, R.G. (1991). Identifying pleasant activities for Alzheimer's disease patients: The Pleasant Events Schedule-AD. *Gerontologist, 21*(1), 124–127.

Vinton, L. (1992). Services planned in abusive elder care situations. *Journal of Elder Abuse and Neglect, 4*(3), 85–99.

Williams, D.P., Wood, E.C., & Moorleghen, F. (1994). An in-service workshop for nursing personnel on the management of catastrophic reactions in dementia victims. *Clinical Gerontologist, 14*(4), 47–54.

6

Role of the
Mental Health Consultant
in Behavior Management

Peter A. Lichtenberg, Ph.D., A.B.P.P., and Susan E. MacNeill, Ph.D.

Mental health consultants perform multiple roles in the assessment and treatment of behavior disturbances in dementia care. These roles include assessing etiology, designing behavioral plans, and coordinating treatment through the interdisciplinary treatment team. This chapter focuses on the first and third roles because the basics of behavior modification and the design of various behavioral plans are covered elsewhere in this volume. Mental health consultants can provide unique skills essential in the development of behavior interventions, including specialized skills in neuropsychology, assessment of depression, and identification of delirium. The following case from the primary author's experience illustrates the need for a combination of careful medical and psychological assessments prior to the development of a behavior intervention.

> While consulting to a 180-bed long-term care facility, staff alerted me to the residents with serious behavior problems. One of my first referrals was to evaluate a man who was "throwing himself to the floor due to manipulative tendencies." In interviewing the staff it was clear that

this man was perceived as falling so as to obtain staff attention. A baseline observation period of 1 day was performed, and we were astounded to note that he fell 31 times. My observations of and interviews with the resident indicated that he often slumped to the floor without warning and lost his balance. In addition, he had severe verbal communication difficulties, was frequently tearful and depressed, had stopped eating, and had lost a considerable amount of weight. At my request this gentleman received comprehensive assessments and treatments in subsequent weeks. A neurologist diagnosed his falls as caused by Parkinson's disease. Consultation with a speech-language pathologist led to the implementation of a Voc-Aid, which greatly improved his ability to communicate. The psychology staff provided counseling to address his depression and a behavior program to increase his social interactions. His depression remitted, and he began to function at a higher level than he had in years. His falling all but disappeared, and he became one of the most social and active residents in the facility.

NEUROPSYCHOLOGY IN LONG-TERM CARE FACILITIES

Behavior problems are elicited by multiple factors, including the person's internal and external environment. Common internal states that cause behavior problems include neuropsychological deficits, depression, and delirium. Neuropsychological assessment, the evaluation of brain–behavior relationships, can yield very useful information regarding diagnosis and treatment of older adults. The following section offers a series of questions to be answered in the assessment process.

Are cognitive deficits present and are they contributing to behavior difficulties?

Many older adults in long-term care experience cognitive deficits associated with cerebral dysfunction. Furthermore, cognitive deficits are a frequent concomitant to behavior management problems. Although neuroimaging techniques are superb indicators of brain dysfunction, they are not useful in identifying a person's functional capacities. In contrast, neuropsychological assessment is useful in determining a person's functional abilities. A neuropsychological assessment can prove invaluable in behavior management by

1. Identifying the level of cognitive deficits present
2. Determining whether cognitive deficits are contributing to behavior difficulties
3. Identifying the pattern of cognitive strengths and weaknesses to assist with treatment planning

Is depression contributing to behavior difficulties?

Depression in older adults may present as social withdrawal, apathy, or agitation, and, consequently, may be recognized initially as a behavior problem. Depression also may have a strong impact on cognition or it may coexist with dementia. Neuropsychological evaluation can aid in the diagnosis of depression. Typically, cognitive deficits solely attributable to depression can be differentiated from progressive dementing illness (Lamberty & Bieliauskas, 1993). More common, however, is the coexistence of dementia and depression, and the behavior disturbance that this condition creates. Frequently, people with dementia become depressed (Rovner, Broadhead, Spencer, Carson, & Folstein, 1989), and this results in additional memory and behavior disorders. When depression is treated adequately, behavior problems often lessen in their intensity or resolve completely. Behavioral treatments for depression in people with dementia lend themselves well to implementation in long-term care facilities because many of the techniques employed can utilize personnel from any number of disciplines. These behavior techniques include engaging the person with dementia in enjoyable activities, the use of social reinforcement, and the use of tangible rewards such as a cup of coffee.

Is delirium contributing to behavior difficulties?

Neuropsychological assessment can help to identify the syndrome of delirium. Identification of delirium is vital because the deficits caused by delirium in people with dementia often are not transitory and can cause further functional decline and higher mortality rates (Francis & Kapoor, 1992; Murray et al., 1993). Thus, early detection of delirium should be emphasized.

ASSESSMENT OF DEMENTIA IN OLDER ADULTS

Traditional neuropsychological assessments have employed standard test batteries such as the Halstead-Reitan Battery. These procedures are extremely lengthy (6–12 hours) and taxing to older adults. Therefore, there is a need in long-term care settings for test batteries to be relatively brief (45–120 minutes) yet diverse in order to assess all general domains of cognitive functioning. Several brief batteries have been developed that can be utilized in dementia evaluations.

WASHINGTON UNIVERSITY TEST BATTERY

One of the first brief test batteries constructed to document the cognitive effects of dementia, the Washington University Test Battery, was part of a longitudinal study of Alzheimer's disease (Storandt, Botwinick, & Danzinger, 1986). The authors utilized portions of the Wechsler Adult Intelligence Scale (WAIS), the Wechsler Memory Scale (WMS), the Benton Visual Retention Test, the Boston

Naming Test, the Trail Making Part A from the Halstead-Reitan Battery, the Bender Gestalt Test, and the Crossing-Off Test in their 90- to 120-minute test battery for dementia evaluations. These tests are paper-and-pencil examinations. Each test contains specific instructions for test administration and scoring. The initial sample included 43 individuals with mild Alzheimer's disease and 43 control subjects enrolled in the Washington University Memory and Aging Project. The subjects were matched on age (mean age, 71 years) and on education (mean educational level, 12.5 years). Follow-up data, collected over a 2.5-year span, were obtained with 22 of the subjects with Alzheimer's disease and 39 of the controls.

Several noteworthy findings came from both the cross-sectional and the longitudinal data. Almost all the tests differentiated the groups initially, including the tests that were hypothesized to be resistant to cerebral deterioration (Information and Comprehension subtests of the WAIS). The Logical Memory subtest of the WMS was the most powerful in distinguishing initially between subjects with Alzheimer's disease and the controls. The only measure that was not useful in distinguishing the groups initially was the Digit Span Forward subtest of the WAIS. Examination of the longitudinal data from this study indicated that, overall, the subjects with Alzheimer's disease deteriorated over the 2½-year-long follow-up period, whereas no change took place in the normal controls.

Although created for research use, this test battery could easily be used in a clinical setting. The battery of tests are diverse enough to tap into multiple domains of cognitive function and yet can detect dementia accurately. The benefits of incorporating this battery would be improved diagnostic accuracy and improved treatment planning, while maintaining a low cost.

CONSORTIUM TO ESTABLISH A REGISTRY FOR ALZHEIMER'S DISEASE (CERAD) TEST BATTERY

In 1989 the 16 National Institutes of Health–designated Alzheimer's disease centers worked together to produce the Consortium to Establish a Registry for Alzheimer's Disease (CERAD) neuropsychological battery (Morris et al., 1989). The aim of the project was to devise a brief 30- to 40-minute-long test battery that would characterize the primary manifestations of Alzheimer's disease. Tests were chosen to represent aspects of memory, language, and praxis. Tests included a verbal fluency test (animal naming); the 15-item Boston Naming Test; the full Mini-Mental State Examination (MMSE); a newly created word list memory task, including delayed recall; and a recognition paradigm and 4 line drawings. In their 1989 paper Morris et al. described the results from 350 subjects with Alzheimer's disease and 275 control subjects. Test-retest reliability correlations over a 1-month period ranged from .52 to .78. The tests readily distinguished normal controls from people with Alzheimer's disease. The authors interpreted these data as providing solid support for the CERAD battery.

Subjects matched for gender, age, and education were utilized in the next investigation of the utility of the CERAD battery. One hundred ninety-six subjects were placed into one of four groups: controls, mildly demented, moderately demented, and severely demented. The average age of the subjects was 71 years, and the average length of education was 14 years. Stepwise linear discriminant function analysis was used to determine how accurately the CERAD battery classified subjects. Of both the controls and the moderately and severely demented groups, 96% were classified accurately, as were 86% of the mildly demented group. The best predictor of cognitive impairment was the delayed recall score from the word list. The percent retained dropped from 85.6% in the controls to 35.8% in the mildly impaired group and to 16% in the moderately and severely impaired groups. The worst predictors were the number of intrusion errors on the word list recall and recognition tasks and the recognition memory score. The authors concluded that the CERAD battery may be useful in aiding in the early detection of dementia. The CERAD battery emphasizes the utility of using psychologists in the evaluation of dementia. The utility of the CERAD battery in answering specific functional referral questions (e.g., ability to live alone) has not been well tested.

NORMATIVE STUDIES RESEARCH PROJECT TEST BATTERY

The Normative Studies Research Project (NSRP) test battery (Lichtenberg, Manning, Vangel, & Ross, 1995) takes between 75 minutes and 2 hours, and emphasizes memory testing. Also included are tests that tap into the domains of language, visuospatial skills, and executive functioning, as well as a test of reading ability. A sampling of 237 older individuals living in an urban area received the following tests: Dementia Rating Scale (DRS), Boston Naming Test, Hooper Visual Organization Test, Visual Form Discrimination Test, and Logical Memory I & II. Of the 237 people studied, 74 were cognitively intact and fully independent in activities of daily living (ADL) abilities, 89 were cognitively impaired and had deficiencies in at least 3 ADLs, and the remaining 73 individuals were either cognitively intact but had ADL deficiencies or cognitively impaired but had few ADL limitations.

Logistic regression analysis was performed to determine the clinical utility of the test battery in classifying people who were not cognitively impaired from people with mild impairment. Because of the high degree of relationship between tests, only the DRS was used. The DRS was a significant predictor of people who were cognitively intact and cognitively impaired ($\chi^2 = 36.03$, $p < .01$), with an overall accurate classification of 75%; sensitivity was at 77% and specificity was at 74%. The DRS had a positive predictive power of 72% and a negative predictive power of 79%. That is, the DRS was relatively better at classifying people with no cognitive impairment than it was in classifying people with cognitive impairment. The data clearly indicate the usefulness of the NSRP test battery for older adults. Relatively good discrimination existed between older adults without cognitive impairment and those with cognitive impairment.

The important benefit of the NSRP battery is its utility with a minority sampling. Studies presented here indicate that, when using appropriate normative data, psychological tests can accurately detect dementia in diverse groups. These data lend credibility to the use of cognitive tests with a broad range of people.

CASE EXAMPLES

The case examples presented in this section offer a framework for evaluating the role of neuropsychological deficits when faced with an older adult's behavior disturbances.

> Mrs. L. was a 73-year-old retired personnel director residing in a long-term care facility who exhibited loud emotional outbursts and experienced auditory hallucinations that resulted in paranoid ideation, verbal accusations, and physical attacks on other residents and staff. She believed that people were plotting to hurt her and were forcing her to go to the bathroom.
>
> **Is there evidence of cerebral impairment?** Mrs. L. was employed as a department head when she began to develop severe problems with alcohol abuse. This abuse caused her to experience a right-hemisphere parieto-occipital stroke. Her medical course was complicated by a 52-day-long coma, grand mal seizures, and high temperatures. She eventually recovered enough cognitive function to return to independent living for 3 years. The loss of a close friend precipitated her admission to a long-term care facility.
>
> **What are the areas of cognitive strengths and weaknesses?** Neuropsychological testing was conducted, and the NSRP test battery revealed moderate to severe cognitive dysfunction, with Mrs. L's visuospatial skills being more impaired than her verbal skills. Basic attention, verbal memory, and reasoning were all relative strengths; visuospatial problem solving, dyspraxia (i.e., a partial loss of the ability to perform skilled, coordinated movements without associated defect in motor or sensory function), and visuospatial memory were all significant weaknesses. Severe left-side sensory and motor deficits were noted.
>
> **How were test results tied to behavior disturbance recommendations?** Deficient visuospatial skills may have caused Mrs. L. to misread facial expressions, and her sensory deficits may have resulted in uncertainty about whether she needed to toilet herself. In treatment of her accusatory behavior, staff were instructed to respond by averting eye contact and to state in a calm voice, "I hear what you have told me." By doing so, Mrs. L's verbal and physical attacks decreased from once a week to three times during a 2-year period.

Mr. C. was a 75-year-old single Caucasian farmer who was admitted to a hospital's acute care unit because he could no longer care for himself. Eight years prior to his hospitalization his family noticed that he was forgetful and confused at times. He began to talk to himself, refused to bathe, and neglected many areas of personal care. The brother with whom Mr. C. lived went away for 2 weeks. Upon his return he found Mr. C. totally disheveled, malnourished, agitated, and wandering. Mr. C. was admitted to a long-term care facility—he weighed 124 pounds, demonstrated anemia, and presented with an agitated depression. His CT scan showed cerebral atrophy. He completed his first neuropsychological assessment 6 weeks later.

Was there evidence of cognitive impairment? On the DRS and MMSE Mr. C's scores were consistent with a rating of severe global cerebral dysfunction. On other tests he scored in the below-average range for general knowledge and in the defective range for verbal abstract reasoning and immediate auditory attention. Mr. C. scored in the severely depressed range on the Geriatric Depression Scale (GDS; see Brink et al., 1982). Mr. C. presented with many severe behavior disorders. He wandered constantly and was intrusive to the point at which he was attacked physically by another resident. He was also extremely restless and moved furniture constantly. Nortriptyline hydrochloride (a drug used to elevate mood) combined with behavioral treatment (described in detail later in the chapter) was used to treat Mr. C's depression, and a low dose of thioridazine hydrochloride (a drug used to reduce agitation) was used to calm him.

What were the cognitive strengths and weaknesses after the depression was treated? Within 6 months Mr. C. demonstrated considerable improvement, particularly in the area of social and affective functioning. His wandering decreased and his intrusiveness subsided. He was no longer depressed, was eating well, was neat and clean, and had gained 20 pounds. Cognitive improvement was also noted, with significant gains in his DRS and MMSE scores. It was found, however, that Mr. C's cognitive abilities were particularly sensitive to physical illness, resulting in delirium. For example, one month he demonstrated a decline in the cognitive screening test results; his score on the MMSE declined significantly. A physical examination revealed that he was dehydrated as a result of his diuretic medication, Lasix (given because he was malnourished). The dosage was reduced and his functioning improved.

What were the practical recommendations? Throughout the final 5 months of his stay at the long-term care facility, Mr. C. continued to demonstrate improvement. Another thorough neuropsychological assessment was performed right before he was discharged. His

DRS score had increased again and was now in the mild-to-moderately impaired range. On tests of word knowledge, attention, and visuospatial abstract reasoning he had improved to the below-average range. Memory was mildly impaired as measured by the Fuld Object Memory Examination. As a result of the improvement in his condition, Mr. C. was discharged to a group home.

Mr. C's case is an example of excess disability secondary to depression and later to delirium in a demented individual. Upon entering long-term care his behavior was typical of residents with advanced Alzheimer's disease. His cognitive abilities were impaired severely and he presented with a myriad of behavior disorders (e.g., wandering, intrusiveness). As his depression and malnutrition were treated he became able to develop trusting relationships with the nursing staff and to improve his eating and grooming abilities. His cognitive abilities steadily improved, and his behavior disturbance disappeared.

ASSESSMENT OF DEPRESSION IN PEOPLE WITH DEMENTIA

Older adults in general, and older people with dementia in particular, present a unique pattern of depressive symptomatology as compared with their younger counterparts. Older people tend to present more commonly with loss of energy, inertia, and extreme withdrawal, rather than florid complaints of mood disorder or suicidal ideation, as reported commonly by younger adults. Perhaps the most useful measure of depression in older adults with mild to moderate levels of dementia is the GDS. In a study of 134 randomly selected individuals four depression instruments were compared for their case-finding abilities in long-term care settings. The GDS emerged as the most successful instrument for detecting depression because of its high sensitivity (Gerety et al., 1994).

BEHAVIORAL THEORY OF DEPRESSION

Lewinsohn and associates' behavioral theory of depression offers a rationale for treatment that is supported by a series of empirical studies. The theory characterizes the maintenance of depression as "a series of person–environment interactions characterized by a deficit in positive experiences and an excess of aversive ones" (Teri & Gallagher-Thompson, 1991, p. 414). In other words, a person's depression is maintained by experiencing an excess of unpleasant events and a lack of pleasant ones.

Since the 1970s Lewinsohn and colleagues have provided empirical support for their theory. Lewinsohn and Graf (1973) presented preliminary data that showed that for young, middle-age, and older adults, pleasant events were significantly related to mood. Lewinsohn and Talkington (1979) created the 160-

item Pleasant Events Schedule for all age groups, which demonstrated reliability and validity. Teri and Lewinsohn (1982) then adapted this scale to older adults, and later, Teri and Logsdon (1991) adapted the scale for people with dementia. In all of the studies mentioned here, pleasant activities were related significantly to depression measures such that the greater the number of pleasant events reported, the lower the level of depression was reported.

BEHAVIORAL TREATMENT WITHIN EXISTING THERAPIES

Lichtenberg, Kimbarow, Morris, and Vangel's (1996) adaptation of the Lewinsohnian model of behavioral treatment of depression is unique in that nonmental health professionals serve as the primary source of that treatment, which comprises the following components: relaxing, mood monitoring, scheduling of pleasant events, and reinforcing functional gains made. In Lichtenberg et al.'s validity study, trained occupational therapists were used to treat depression in both older adults who were cognitively intact and those who had mild to moderate dementia (mean age, 77 years) in a geriatric rehabilitative setting. This method of treatment was found to be highly effective in reducing symptoms of depression and was associated with high levels of resident satisfaction with the treatment program. The adaptation of the Lewinsohnian behavioral treatment model by the primary author and his associates is designed to occur concomitantly with other standard treatment courses, such as occupational, physical, speech-language, or recreational therapy sessions in a rehabilitation program or a long-term care setting.

In order to maintain an acceptable degree of consistency in each depression treatment session it is necessary to establish an individualized standard approach for each older adult. This approach ensures that any differences in outcome can be attributed to factors that are most likely beyond the control of the clinician and facilitates a valid quantitative analysis of outcome. For example, an individual's mood may be influenced by his or her success or failure during regular occupational therapy. If his or her mood was measured on some days after therapy and on other days after administration of the Pleasant Events Schedule, a level of uncertainty to the outcome would be added. Lichtenberg and co-workers recommend that the length of the individualized therapy session be 45–90 minutes. During the first 20 minutes and the last 20 minutes of each session, the therapist should conduct a variety of behavioral treatment interventions. The session should be organized as follows (detailed methods for this approach are described by Lichtenberg et al., 1995):

Rating individual's mood
Administering relaxation treatment
Scheduling pleasant events
Rating individual's mood

Setting goals
Conducting occupational therapy treatment
Graphing progress
Rating individual's mood

ASSESSMENT OF DELIRIUM IN OLDER ADULTS

Like dementia and depression, delirium is a term that describes a syndrome. A syndrome is a constellation of behaviors that has any number of etiologies (i.e., sources). The criteria for delirium have been simplified in the *Diagnostic and Statistical Manual of Mental Disorders-IV* (American Psychological Association, 1994). They include a disturbance of consciousness and change in cognition that develops over a short period of time and fluctuates throughout the day. Trzepacz, Baker, and Greenhouse (1987) developed the Delirium Rating Scale for use by mental health consultants. The mental health consultant interviews the resident and nursing staff to assess 10 areas of resident functioning during the previous 24 hours. These areas include the following:

1. Temporal onset; by definition, delirium has an abrupt onset
2. Perceptual disturbance; visual illusions and the inability to discriminate well between dreams and reality are symptoms associated with delirium
3. Hallucination type; auditory, visual, and/or tactile hallucinations are possible in people with delirium
4. Delusions; in delirium, delusions are new and poorly organized and thus quite different from the delusions of, for example, a person with paranoid schizophrenia, which occur over a long period of time and are quite specific
5. Psychomotor behavior; delirium in older adults most commonly presents as hypoactive behaviors (e.g., withdrawal, lethargy), but also can present as hyperactive behaviors (e.g., agitation, combativeness) or a fluctuation between hypo- and hyperactive behaviors
6. Cognitive decline; an essential part of the diagnosis of delirium and includes deterioration, even in people with dementia
7. Lability of mood, changing from happiness to sadness or from inhibition to disinhibition
8. The resident's sleep–wake cycle is often disrupted with delirium; notable variations in level of arousal or alertness are common
9. Variability of symptoms, with a waxing and waning of symptoms, is common to delirium
10. Physical disorders are the most likely cause of delirium, including drug, infection, metabolic, medication, or a new-onset central nervous system disorder

Delirium is most common in older adults with dementia (Erkinjuntti, Wilkstrom, Paolo, & Autio, 1986; Rockwood, 1993). In Erkinjuntti and associates' study of 2,000 consecutive admissions to departments of medicine for adults older than age 55, for example, the overall prevalence of delirium was 11%. When only older people with dementia were examined in the sample, however, the prevalence rose to 41%. Rockwood's prospective study in a geriatric assessment unit found the chief causes of delirium to be medications (31%), infection (23%), congestive heart failure (21%), and metabolic disorders (19%). Thus, all clinicians must learn more about the rapid identification of delirium, particularly with frail older adults.

ORGANIZATIONAL ISSUES IN LONG-TERM CARE FACILITIES

Understanding the organizational aspects of a long-term care team is critical in order for mental health consultants' knowledge of behavioral issues to be effective in long-term care facilities. Without understanding the various aspects of team organization, these consultants will often find themselves ineffective and frustrated. Innovations to improve the quality of geriatric long-term care can occur only when the mental health consultant involves nursing assistants and licensed practical nurses. Licensed practical nurses and nursing assistants hold the majority of full-time positions (88%) and more than half of all positions in geriatric long-term care (Kasteler, Ford, White, & Carruth, 1979; Smyer, Cohn, & Brannon, 1988). Nursing assistants outnumber licensed practical nurses 4:1 and licensed practical nurses outnumber registered nurses 1.5:1. Two studies provided insight as to how nursing assistants and licensed practical nurses spend their time (Burgio, Engel, Hawkins, McCormick, & Scheve, 1990): Providing resident care and interacting with residents were the predominant activities, and for the most part, the staff were rated as treating their residents as equals.

It is thus remarkable to realize that, although they provide most of the care to residents, nursing assistants in particular are discouraged from verbalizing their ideas about resident care and are not even considered an active part of the interdisciplinary health care team (Faulkner, 1985; Kasteler et al., 1979; Sbordone & Sterman, 1983; Schwartz, 1974; Smith, Discenza, & Saxberg, 1978; Stein, Linn, & Elliot, 1986). Thus, although nursing assistants are heavily involved in difficult resident care, they often feel isolated and neglected.

Turnover among nursing assistants is high, is costly to the institution, and has considerable effect on the quality of care provided (Kasteler et al., 1979; Schwartz, 1974; Smyer et al., 1988; Waxman & Carner, 1984). Kasteler et al. and Schwartz reported turnover of nursing assistants at 75% per year, whereas, among seven long-term care facilities, Waxman and Carner found it to vary from 5% to 76% per year. Kasteler et al. interviewed 426 terminated nursing assistants in order to identify the problems they encountered. A majority of the nursing assistants were disenchanted with the understaffing and overwork with which they coped, along with organizational problems such as poor supervision and communication. Waxman et al. concluded that a rigid organizational structure, one that did not allow the nursing assistants to communicate with professional staff, was a major contributor to turnover. Smith et al. (1978) found that 71% of the nursing assistants and licensed practical nurses had contact with the director of nursing only through their charge nurses.

Successful programming, such as can be provided by mental health consultants, often hinges on whether the organizational climate can change as well. In reviewing successful efforts, Sbordone and Sterman (1983) reported that increased communication among hierarchies of staff led to reduced turnover and improved staff morale. Chartock, Nevins, Rzetelny, and Gilberto (1988) were able to increase the time staff could spend to bathe residents so that emotional as well as physical needs could be attended to, and they were able to include nursing assistants in the treatment team meetings.

INTERDISCIPLINARY TEAM ISSUES IN LONG-TERM CARE FACILITIES

Often, psychologists who are not accustomed to working within a health care team dynamic are overwhelmed by long-term care practices. Interdisciplinary teams have long been hailed in health care as the best way to deliver care despite the fact that few methodologically sound studies have been performed on team care (Halstead, 1976). In addition, the experiences of some clinicians and teams are quite sobering (Bates-Smith & Tsukuda, 1984; De Santis, 1983). De Santis found that team members from a long-term care facility spent their time vying for influence over the team rather than focusing on resident goals and that team meetings were routinely boycotted. Bates-Smith and Tsukuda reported that, too often, value differences and role confusions deter the team from functioning properly. These studies are useful in that they illustrate the necessity to plan team interactions and to build team cohesiveness.

To be an effective interdisciplinary team member, mental health consultants working in long-term care settings must recognize the different models of functioning from which various team members operate. For instance, Brown and Zimberg (1982) and Qualls and Czirr (1988) focused on the differences between the medical and psychosocial models. In the diagnostic process, for instance, the medical model uses a "ruling out," or determining one etiology approach, whereas the psychosocial model uses a "ruling in," or at least acknowledging the effects of a variety of factors (e.g., loss, health, stress, depression). Medical practitioners are usually paternalistic with older adult residents and concerned with immediate results, versus psychosocial practitioners, who view the resident more as a partner and use slower methods of assessment. The differences in these models may lead to conflicts among practitioners on a team. The practitioner must both understand the models of functioning brought by other team members and make oneself understood.

Involving nursing assistants in the meetings of the interdisciplinary team is not enough to improve communication; the mental health consultant must provide them with support and training. Assertiveness training is helpful because it provides nursing assistants with a tool for communicating their concerns about resident care. Training in some basic aspects of dementia, depression and loss, and team functioning is also useful. If administrative support is available, psychologists can be instrumental in forming and leading support groups for nursing assistants (Lichtenberg, 1994). Finally, mental health consultants must demonstrate flexibility and change behavioral plans when they no longer work. The following case example underscores the involvement of team members that is required to improve behaviors in residents and the flexibility that is needed to maintain those improvements.

At age 7 Mrs. M. was abandoned by her parents and went to live with an aunt who severely abused her, often banging Mrs. M's head against a wall. As a teenager Mrs. M. married a man 20 years her senior. He beat her regularly, often striking her about the head. At age 30 damage to her brain caused her to feel a burning sensation, as well as numbness, weakness, pain, and depression. Mrs. M. was given an intellectual assessment and her score placed her in the range "mild mental retardation." Her verbal skills were better than her visuospatial skills, and attention was a strength, whereas problem solving was a prominent deficit. At age 65 Mrs. M. was admitted to long-term care because she displayed severe agitation and bouts of crying. She exhibited long periods of yelling at others and accusing them of harming her. Her psychiatric diagnosis was organic mood syndrome, indicating brain damage that was not specified as to location.

Mrs. M. complained constantly of abuse by staff members. She slept poorly, screamed often, and attacked other residents. Trying desperately to appease her, staff gave in to her requests for three whirlpool baths per day: Inadvertently, staff were rewarding the outbursts. It was at this point that the nursing assistants brought Mrs. M's problems to the attention of the facility's mental health consultant. The consultant's behavioral treatment goals were to reduce Mrs. M's outbursts and to increase her prosocial behavior.

The interdisciplinary team met after the completion of a psychological consultation and agreed to institute the behavior technique of differential reinforcement of other behaviors. The target behaviors selected were loud yelling, crying, or hitting. Initially, Mrs. M. had the opportunity to earn small rewards (e.g., coffee, telephone call to family, manicure) in three 1-hour periods each day. If in one week she earned 13 small rewards, she was given a large reward (e.g., trip to town, trip to snack bar). During the next week the reward periods increased by 15 minutes, thus demanding more from Mrs. M., but using the same type of reward system. At all times, if Mrs. M. screamed or hit others, she was placed in time-out for 30 minutes. Her behavior improved steadily. By 6 months her screaming incidents had declined by 50% and her hitting had fallen by 80%. By 12 months she no longer struck anyone, and incidents of screaming were rare.

Twenty months into the plan, however, Mrs. M. began to demonstrate screaming and crying regularly—the intervention plan was no longer working. The rewards had lost their potency, and observation of Mrs. M. revealed that arguing with staff on the way to time-out was now rewarding. Armed with quantitative data, the nursing assistants directly asked the mental health consultant to develop a new care program. Soon after, the mental health consultant introduced a plan calling for nonexclusionary time-out. Mrs. M. was given a corsage to wear when she was calm and quiet. When wearing the corsage, she received verbal praise and social reinforcers. When Mrs. M. began to yell, curse, or make accusations of others, the corsage was taken and Mrs. M. was ignored and excluded from all activities. Every 15 minutes thereafter, staff would check to see if Mrs. M. was quiet; if she was quiet, she received her corsage. The only time the care plan was to be interrupted was for medical reasons or emergencies.

The plan did not show much promise during its first 4 months. However, gains came rapidly thereafter. Mrs. M. demonstrated appropriate behavior for 2 weeks until, for reasons unknown, she spent much of one day yelling. At the next interdisciplinary team meeting the licensed practical nurse asked that Mrs. M's plan be dropped because she felt that it was not working. The quantitative data gathered by the team showed that, in fact, Mrs. M's plan was working, so it was retained. During the next 60 days Mrs. M. lost her corsage only once and only briefly.

Mrs. M's case highlights several essential components of behavior management: First, it shows the importance of achieving staff consensus before embarking on an ambitious plan because lasting success comes slowly. Second, no care plan works forever—teams must demonstrate flexibility in their treatment efforts. Third, quantitative data must be obtained in order to evaluate treatment. In Mrs. M's case quantitative data identified when the plan was working and when it was no longer useful, whereas qualitative data (i.e., staff perceptions) were vulnerable to bias and false conclusions. Finally, this case demonstrates that teams can have a positive impact on even the most difficult behavior problems.

SUMMARY

The role of the mental health consultant in the treatment of behavior disorders in older adults with dementia is to broaden the assessment and treatment expertise of the interdisciplinary team. Before the team launches into a time-intensive behavior modification program, mental health consultants can provide valuable data on the resident's functioning. Specifically the consultant can determine how the person's neuropsychological status, including the delineation of cognitive strengths and weaknesses and the assessment of depression and of delirium, may affect the behavior disturbance. Depending on the specifics of these findings, the mental health consultant may recommend various approaches to treatment, such as the ones described earlier in the chapter.

The mental health consultant serves an equally important role in helping the treatment team to function better. By being attuned to both organizational issues (e.g., communication) and team training needs (mainly information based), the mental health consultant can enhance the likelihood of success of treatments for behavior disturbance. The consultant is encouraged to view his or her roles broadly and attempt to incorporate mental health expertise in a number of geriatric and health care issues.

CONCLUSION

This chapter describes the utility of cognitive and affective assessment, as behavior disorders often can be best understood within the context of cognitive abilities and cerebral dysfunction. Specific case examples as well as brief test batteries are presented herein. In addition, the importance of assessing for delirium is examined. The latter portion of the chapter reviews the importance of understanding the organizational climate within long-term care facilities. Tips are included so as to enhance the role of nursing assistants and improve the quality of the mental health consultation.

REFERENCES

American Psychological Association. (1994). *Diagnostic and statistical manual of mental disorders* (4th ed.). Washington, DC: Author.

Bates-Smith, K., & Tsukuda, R.A. (1984). Problems of an interdisciplinary training team. *Clinical Gerontologist, 3,* 66–68.

Brink, T., Yesavage, J., Lum, G., Heersema, P., Addey, M., & Rose, T. (1982). Screening tests for geriatric depression. *Clinical Gerontologist, 1,* 37–41.

Brown, H.N., & Zimberg, N.E. (1982). Difficulties in the integration of psychological and medical practices. *American Journal of Psychiatry, 139,* 1576–1580.

Burgio, L.D., Engel, B.T., Hawkins, A., McCormick, K., & Scheve, A. (1990). Descriptive analysis of nursing staff behaviors in a teaching nursing home: Differences among NAs, LPNs, and RNs. *Gerontologist, 30,* 107–112.

Chartock, P., Nevins, A., Rzetelny, H., & Gilberto, P. (1988). A mental health training program in nursing homes. *Gerontologist, 28,* 503–507.

De Santis, G. (1983). From teams to hierarchy: A short-lived innovation in a hospital for the elderly. *Social Science Medicine, 17,* 1613–1618.

Erkinjuntti, T., Wilkstrom, J., Paolo, J., & Autio, L. (1986). Dementia among medical inpatients. *Archives of Internal Medicine, 146,* 1923–1926.

Faulkner, A.O. (1985). Interdisciplinary health care teams: An educational approach to improvement of health care for the aged. *Gerontology and Geriatrics Education, 5,* 29–39.

Francis, J., & Kapoor, W. (1992). Prognosis after hospital discharge of older adult medical patients with delirium. *Journal of the American Geriatrics Society, 40,* 601–606.

Gerety, M.B., Williams, J.W., Mulrow, C.D., Cornell, J.E., Kadri, A.A., Rosenberg, J., Chiodo, L.K., & Long, M. (1994). Performance of case-finding tools for depression in the nursing home. Influence of clinical and functional characteristics and selection of optimal threshold scores. *Journal of the American Geriatrics Society, 42,* 1103–1109.

Halstead, L.S. (1976). Team care in chronic illness: A critical review of the literature of the past 25 years. *Archives of Physical Medicine and Rehabilitation, 57,* 507–511.

Kasteler, J.M., Ford, M.H., White, M.A., & Carruth, M.L. (1979). Personnel turnover: A major problem for nursing homes. *Nursing Homes, 28,* 20–27.

Lamberty, G.J., & Bieliauskas, L.A. (1993). Distinguishing between depression and dementia in the elderly: A review of neuropsychological findings. *Archives of Clinical Neuropsychology, 8,* 149–170.

Lewinsohn, P.M., & Graf, M. (1973). Pleasant activities and depression. *Journal of Consulting and Clinical Psychology, 41,* 261–268.

Lewinsohn, P., & Talkington, J. (1979). Studies in the measurement of unpleasant life events and relations with depression. *Applied Psychological Measurement, 3,* 83–101.

Lichtenberg, P.A. (1994). *A guide to psychological practice in geriatric long term care.* Binghamton, NY: Haworth Press.

Lichtenberg, P.A., Kimbarow, M.L., Morris, P., & Vangel, S.J. (1996). Behavioral treatment of depression in predominantly African American medical patients. *Clinical Gerontologist, 17,* 15–33.

Lichtenberg, P.A., Manning, C.A., Vangel, S.J., & Ross, T.P. (1995). Normative and ecological validity data in older urban medical patients: A program of neuropsychological research. *Advances in Medical Psychotherapy, 8,* 121–136.

Morris, J.C., Heyman, A., Mohs, R.C., Hughes, J.P., vanBelle, G., Fillenbaum, G., et al. (1989). Consortium to Establish a Registry for Alzheimer's Disease (CERAD). *Neurology, 39,* 1159–1165.

Murray, A.M., Levkoff, S.E., Wetle, T.T., Becket, L., Cleary, P.D., Schor, J.D., Lipsitz, L.A., Rowe, J.W., & Evans, D.A. (1993). Acute delirium and functional decline in the hospitalized elderly patient. *Journal of Gerontology: Medical Sciences, 48,* M181–M186.

Qualls, S.H., & Czirr, R. (1988). Geriatric health teams: Classifying models of professional and team functioning. *Gerontologist, 28,* 372–376.

Rockwood, K. (1993). The occurrence and duration of symptoms in elderly patients with delirium. *Journal of Gerontology: Medical Sciences, 48,* M162–M166.

Rovner, B.W., Broadhead, J., Spencer, M., Carson, K., & Folstein, M. (1989). Depression and Alzheimer's disease. *American Journal of Psychiatry, 146,* 350–353.

Sbordone, R.J., & Sterman, L.T. (1983). The psychologist as a consultant in a nursing home: Effect on staff morale and turnover. *Professional Psychology, 14,* 240–250.

Schwartz, A. (1974). Staff development and morale building in nursing homes. *Gerontologist, 14,* 50–54.

Smith, H.L., Discenza, R., & Saxberg, B.O. (1978). Administering long-term care services: A decision-making perspective. *Gerontologist, 18,* 159–166.

Smyer, M., Cohn, M., & Brannon, D. (1988). *Mental health consultation in nursing homes.* New York: New York University Press.

Stein, S., Linn, M.W., & Elliot, E.M. (1986). The relationship between nursing home residents' perceptions of nursing staff and quality of nursing home care. *Journal of Physical and Occupational Therapy, 4,* 143–156.

Storandt, M., Botwinick, J., & Danzinger, W.L. (1986). Longitudinal changes: Patients with mild SDAT and matched healthy controls. In L.W. Poon (Ed.), *Clinical memory assessment of older adults.* Washington, DC: American Psychological Association.

Teri, L., & Gallagher-Thompson, D. (1991). Cognitive-behavior interventions for treatment of depression in Alzheimer patients. *Gerontologist, 31,* 413–416.

Teri, L., & Lewinsohn, P. (1982). Modification of the pleasant and unpleasant events schedules for use with the elderly. *Journal of Consulting and Clinical Psychology, 50,* 444–445.

Teri, L., & Logsdon, R.G. (1991). Identifying pleasant activities for Alzheimer disease patients: The Pleasant Events Schedule-AD. *Gerontologist, 31,* 124–127.

Trzepacz, P.T., Baker, R.W., & Greenhouse, J. (1987). A symptom rating scale for delirium. *Psychiatry Research, 23,* 89–97.

Waxman, H.M., & Carner, E.A. (1984). Physicians' recognition, diagnosis, and treatment of mental disorders in elderly medical patients. *Gerontologist, 24,* 593–597.

7

Family and Staff—
Partners in Caregiving

Kathleen C. Buckwalter, Ph.D., R.N., F.A.A.N.; Marianne Smith, R.N., M.S.;
Meridean Maas, Ph.D., R.N., F.A.A.N.; and Lisa Kelley, R.N., M.A.

Transfer of a loved one with dementia from home to a nursing facility is a diffi-cult transition for many family[1] members. Often, the family member has cared for the person with dementia for a long period of time in his or her home. When the difficult decision is made that care can no longer be provided at home and the person with dementia is relocated, the family caregiver experiences a sudden and drastic change in role: No longer is the family member the primary caregiver who has control over the care of the relative with dementia. Suddenly, the family care-giver feels he or she is the outsider, with no legitimate or sanctioned caregiving role within the confines of the long-term care institution. This change can be con-

Supported in part by Grant No. RO1-NR01689, The Family Involvement in Care grant, funded by the National Institute of Nursing Research, Meridean Maas, Ph.D., R.N., and Elizabeth Swanson, Ph.D., R.N., coprincipal investigators.

[1]The word "family" means all the people who are important to the resident and who play a significant role in the resident's life—immediate family members (spouse, children), old friends or neighbors, "adopted" (e.g., saying "she's like a daughter to me") children, or actual relatives.

fusing and stressful for many caregivers; they may not know how to continue their caregiving role. The result may be family member complaints such as, "There's no place for us to visit . . . there's no privacy" "His dentures are missing—again!" "It's always too cold in Mom's room!" "The laundry ruined Dad's favorite shirt!" or "She's never properly dressed when I come to take her on an outing" on a regular basis (Smith, Buckwalter, & Mitchell, 1993).

When staff are doing their best to provide good-quality care to residents, family and other loved ones' complaints and accusations often seem unfair and hurtful, and can make staff angry. One way staff can circumvent these feelings is by asking themselves, "Why is this happening? What is *really* going on here?" By understanding families' behavior, staff can learn to respond in ways that defuse the situation and help to prevent or solve problems before family members become angry, frustrated, or both. Understanding families' feelings and behaviors also helps staff to focus on the development of cooperative relationships with families rather than the troublesome or threatening aspects of families' actions.

This chapter examines the relationship between family members and nursing facility caregivers. It describes how long-term care staff can respond best to family members when they are difficult, demanding, or otherwise unpleasant, and explains some of the mixed feelings that staff hold about families of the residents with whom they work. The final section of the chapter is an in-depth look at the Family Involvement in Care (FIC) protocol, a family–staff partnership intervention designed to help nursing facility staff and family members work together to provide the best care for the families' loved ones, the residents with dementia (Maas, Buckwalter, Swanson, Specht, Tripp-Reimer, & Hardy, 1994; Maas & Swanson, 1991). This information is key because both families and staff are important components of the nursing facility environment and integral to a good quality of life for the resident. Indeed, interacting with residents' families is a significant, though often devalued, part of staff members' jobs (Maas, Buckwalter, Kelley, & Stolley, 1991). Some of the ways that families are important include the following (Morris & Murphy, 1995):

- Providing the resident with a link to the past and to life outside the nursing facility
- Providing staff with a wealth of historical and current information about the resident
- Helping to oversee care, in order to maintain optimal quality
- Helping staff with activities the resident enjoys
- Providing socialization and affection
- Helping celebrate special events, such as birthdays, Christmas, or Hanukkah
- Actually assisting staff as caregivers

Moreover, stress among either family members or staff can contribute to resident distress, exacerbating agitation and other problem behaviors associated with dementia (Maas et al., 1994). Thus, better understanding of families and their needs can help staff to improve resident care and ease otherwise difficult aspects of their own jobs.

FAMILIES: AN IMPORTANT BUT NEGLECTED RESOURCE

Families are a neglected resource in most long-term care facilities (Buckwalter & Hall, 1987). They can help both their loved ones and other residents in a variety of ways such as providing direct care, offering support and encouragement, and brightening the day with kind words or good deeds. With encouragement, support, and permission to do so, families can play an even larger and more welcome role in most facilities. Families can make staff members' work less stressful. Conversely, if family members have personality conflicts with staff members and are uncomfortable with or uncertain about the roles they should play in the long-term care setting, even the best care plans may not be executed. As one family member noted (Kelley, 1997),

> They [staff] asked me what I expected of them and I said, "I expect her to be taken care of and I absolutely will not put up with any mental or physical abuse and other than that I don't know what to tell you." Because we didn't abuse my mother and we didn't intend to have any mental abuse there either. Because some of them can be like that. There's some of them that just aren't cut out to be an aide or a nurse, especially on the Alzheimer's unit.

As mentioned earlier, in order to respond appropriately when family members become upset, staff need to better understand what causes this behavior. Most often, the behavior has an antecedent, a cause. Staff must find the chain of events that led up to the family's angry, frustrated, or demanding behavior. If staff understand the causes of family behavior, they will be better able to help families cope with the stress of role change, enlist the families' help with caregiving, and prevent frustration, anger, and conflicts with staff.

COMMON SOURCES OF STRESS

Placing a loved one with dementia in a nursing facility is an enormously stressful event (Wilson, 1989). Although each family is different, common stresses tend to recur in all placements. These stresses include (Smith et al., 1993)

- Long-standing patterns of relating to one another and problems between family members that follow residents into the facility
- Stress created by changes in the family's structure and the way that the family interacts and relates to one another after placement of the person with dementia
- Problems and stresses at home that have little or nothing to do with the resident, except that they compete for the family member's time and attention

- Stresses of caregiving prior to the placement that can affect the mental health of the family caregiver
- Stress of the actual placement process, which is influenced strongly by both family and cultural values

These stressors are illustrated by the comments made by two adult children who are caregivers regarding their siblings (Kelley, 1997):

He's [brother] worthless in terms of he doesn't help. He doesn't come up and come see her.

I go see her more than any of the family. My brother comes up from out of town and I have to push him, or I have to go and get her and bring her [to my house] so he can see her. And I'm sorry if he's uncomfortable in the nursing facility, but she's his mother, for goodness sake.

It is important for staff to remember that the resident's adult children likely have their own families. Middle-age women, in particular, are often pegged as belonging to the "sandwich generation," because they are caught [or sandwiched] between the demands of their own children and those of caring for an aging parent, with people in both age groups needing their time, attention, energy, and financial support (Brody, 1985). Also, increasingly, other older family members have their own limitations or illnesses to manage. A loved one's placement in a nursing facility may require them to take on responsibilities that are unfamiliar, unwanted, and uncomfortable. Furthermore, these older family members likely have fewer resources to call on to support them through this stressful period. For example, lack of money, poor health, and lack of transportation may cause family stresses postplacement.

Staff must consider what family members coped with before the resident was admitted to the facility. The caregiving experience itself may have had a negative impact on their mental health and social and economic resources. Indeed, the stresses of caregiving are linked consistently to increased physical illness, depression, substance abuse, social isolation, and physical abuse among family caregivers (George & Gwyther, 1986). Many times, at the point when a care recipient enters a nursing facility, family caregivers are emotionally and physically exhausted, as demonstrated by an adult daughter's comments (Kelley, 1997):

Oh, it's [care] so much better because I couldn't take care of Mother at home. The patience it would take! I love her dearly, but 24 hours a day! I wouldn't get any sleep. I couldn't have any normal life with my own children. At home, it would be dreadful.

Too often, family members delay a loved one's placement in long-term care until they can no longer cope with caregiving duties. They wait until the care recipients are completely unable to care for themselves, when there is not enough time, energy, or outside assistance available to care properly for loved ones with dementia at home. It is not surprising, then, that some family members cannot summon the energy to be helpful to or understanding of the nursing facility staff (Kelley, 1997):

> I don't think everybody's cut out to take care of those people [older people with dementia]. . . . You have to be really strong. I found out in the apartment that I weakened as time went on. I tried to be strong but it was weakening . . . just wearing me down.

As stated earlier, usually families do not abandon their caregiving roles with the admission of their loved ones to a long-term care facility (Max, Webber, & Fox, 1995). Rather, the nature of family involvement in care changes when the person with dementia enters a dementia-specific care unit (DSCU) or nursing facility (Bowers, 1988; Duncan & Morgan, 1994). Although family members may feel relieved to have made the placement decision, they may be trying to cope with many unresolved emotions as well. In some cases families may view the nursing facility itself as a "place to go to die," "like being in jail," or "a fate worse than death." Thus, the decision to place a family member in a nursing facility is likely to arouse intense and often negative feelings (Stephens, Kinney, & Ogrocki, 1991; Zarit & Whitlatch, 1992). As two family members put it (Kelley, 1997)

> I tell you, if I lived in a nursing facility, I'd run to the furthermost corner of my imagination and stay there. I wouldn't try to come out and take part in it either.

> I was really surprised that the nursing facility didn't turn out to be the "house of horrors" that I thought it would.

COMMON EMOTIONAL REACTIONS

The transition process may arouse many emotions in family members and in their loved ones with dementia. They may experience intense feelings of sadness and loss, anger, disappointment, or even resentment. Some people may feel guilty, believing that they, or others, should have been able to "do more" to prevent institutionalization. Others worry about how the move will affect them and their loved ones, and still others are anxious about resorting to long-term care placement, as in the following example (Kelley, 1997):

> Well, see, my husband wonders why do I come down here because Dad doesn't really know us and stuff . . . to me it's seeing if his needs seem to be met. . . . You have to think for them. And since the individual family knows more of the history, like his stomach is a problem. Or that medication to him is stronger than to normal people . . . we know that, and the staff, they've got 30 other people to keep track of. Where I think our role is is to be kind of his eyes and ears. . . . As he's getting worse and worse, you have to do more of that. You have to be more on the ball because he can't do it for himself. . . . I mean, I just can't see abandoning him . . .

Family members may feel guilty, ashamed, or that they are abandoning their spouse or parents. Many adult children wrestle with the dilemma of what "honor thy father and mother" means in terms of providing care, and they do much soul searching about their personal responsibilities for caring for an aging parent. One daughter commented, "She [Mom] was always there for us, we'll always be there for her" (Kelley, 1997). These beliefs and attitudes affect both the decisions that families make and how stressful the consequences are for them. To compound the difficulty of this situation, care recipients may interpret family members' genuine inability to provide care as unwillingness to meet their obligations and, as a result, may feel unloved and abandoned (e.g., feelings such as "Where are they when I need them?").

Many families experience all of the emotions mentioned above; there are no rules about what or when people feel. Some family members may feel the most disturbed at the time that their loved one is placed in a long-term care facility, whereas others become more upset the longer their loved one resides in the facility.

Staff must be aware of and control their own emotions when working with upset residents and/or their families. Lack of emotional control puts them at risk for becoming part of a family power struggle, sidestepping the person or the problem, becoming upset and angry themselves, or reacting in a way that causes the situation to deteriorate further. As with other types of problems, prevention is the best medicine (Smith et al., 1993). Staff can prevent difficulties if they make sure that families know they have been listened to, taken seriously, and given opportunities to interact with staff or administrators. The alternative can be problematic, as noted in the following statements from family members (Kelley, 1997):

> I feel good coming up here and having staff call me by name. It's sort of become a second home for me . . . but the top level just walk right by and never say good morning to my good morning, don't smile till I smile, and I find that disconcerting.

> No one has ever said anything to me. My husband wondered if they wanted me to really be there as much as I am . . . but I don't feel like I'm doing anything wrong.

FAMILY ASSESSMENT

Family assessment focuses on the type and level of stress that family members experience, and on the caregiver–care recipient relationship prior to placement in a DSCU. Early recognition that family members are having difficulty coping may help staff ease the family's fear or guilt and prevent them from becoming frustrated or angry. It is also important for staff to gather as much background information on the family and resident as possible. Too often, staff do not know what was said, what kind of promises were made, who was involved in the decision to place the family member in a DSCU, or even what kind of relationship the resident had with his or her family prior to admission—all of which can influence resident and family behavior. Situations such as that described in the following can have a significant impact on the resident in question (Kelley, 1997):

Nobody else would bother with him. My children didn't want to bother with him. He was not very nice to them . . . as they were growing up. He physically abused one of them. And the others he just ignored. Just had no association with them at all. Nothing. So, this is why my children do not go down to visit him. They can't forgive him. And I'm not asking them to either. They are all adults. They know what they need to do.

In a family assessment, facility staff must assess their own contributions to problem behavior. A staff member should ask him- or herself honestly, Do I really listen or pay attention? How well do I communicate with family members/the person with dementia? What am I doing that might be making the family or the person with dementia upset? Have I neglected to do the things the family has asked me to do? Is any part of their concern valid?

INTERVENTIONS WITH FAMILIES

Staff can use two general approaches—both of which demand time and skill—to defuse problems with families (Smith et al., 1993): The first approach is for staff to respond in appropriate ways to the families' feelings, whether anger, sadness, guilt, fear, or some other emotion. Staff who verbalize the emotional distress that family members experience and support their right to feel negative feelings often help family members feel better through emotional crisis intervention and sympathetic statements such as, "This must be a pretty rough time for you. Lots of family members feel sad or guilty about placing their loved one in a nursing facility, and those feelings are pretty understandable, given all the stress that you've been under. This is a difficult, and even frightening, situation to face." To best support family members who are upset, staff should

- Be nonjudgmental: accept that family members feel the way that they do, even when their negative expressions or emotions are directed at the residents or the staff
- Explain how sadness, guilt, and other "negative" emotions are natural responses to the decision to place a family member in a DSCU
- Encourage family members to talk or cry openly while listening and provide nonverbal support (e.g., eye contact, gentle touch)

The second approach is for staff to work with family members to find solutions to perceived problems. Staff should help family members rethink the situation and solicit the help of family members in solving care problems. For example, staff can (Schwartz & Vogel, 1990)

- Remind family members of all of the positive things they have done to support the resident, both in the past and at present

- Provide ways in which family members can support the resident now that he or she is living in the nursing facility
- Educate family members about dementia: how it will affect their loved one and what staff are doing to care for the person with the disease
- Encourage involvement in support and/or community groups, in activities within the nursing facility, or with friends/family members of other residents
- Suggest other activities or outlets (e.g., encouraging family members to bring in mementos or items of importance to the resident)

Staff should not personalize the problem and become angry themselves or argue with family members and become defensive. They should remember that family viewpoints are not always rational. Also, staff should not minimize the conflict. Finally, staff must keep in mind that they may be a convenient target for anger, and not the cause of the problem. Responses that can help to defuse the anger or upset that family members express include the following (Smith et al., 1993):

- Accepting that they are angry/upset and encouraging them to express their feelings
- Listening carefully to what is being said in order to figure out what the problem is without taking sides, arguing, or offering advice
- Asking questions in order to clarify information
- Restating the problem and narrowing its scope to address only the issues that are relevant to the facility
- Discussing the expectations held by family members and what the staff can reasonably deliver
- Following through with what staff agreed to do (e.g., reporting the problem to another staff member or administrator in order to arrive at a solution; acknowledging an error or oversight and apologizing to the family member[s]; controlling their own emotions by leaving the room, calming down, thinking about the problem, and joining the family member at a later time)

In working toward a solution, staff must accept the fact that a family member has a problem with them or the facility, even when they do not perceive the family's complaint as a "real problem." The more information that staff provide to family members and the more they involve family in making decisions about caregiving, the more control family members feel they have, the more likely they are to find solutions to perceived problems, and the more likely they are to feel positive and support what is done for them, as in the following comments made by family members (Kelley, 1997):

They tell me anything I ask. I can't complain about that a bit.

If anything happens, they call me. If he gets a scratch or falls or whatever . . . they are always good to answer, to tell me what they can.

Once staff have accepted the fact of the family's anger, they should work on a plan for reaching mutual staff and family goals and for communicating the plan to all of the "players"—staff, family members, and residents, if possible—and involve everyone in the planning. Ways to involve family members in this planning are to ask them to watch for and communicate positive changes in the resident (i.e., letting staff know when residents do well) and to assist with care activities that help to resolve the problem (e.g., helping to bathe or feed the resident). In addition to involving family members in finding and implementing a solution to the problem, staff should discuss how long it may take to reach resolution. Most problems do not develop "overnight" and, consequently, cannot be resolved "overnight." Both staff and family members, however, need to feel that they are making progress toward a goal and to evaluate whether the proposed plan, or any part of it, is working. In the care of people with dementia changes sometimes take place in such small increments that staff and family members lose sight of the fact that progress is being made. A good way to help both staff and family members track progress is to schedule regular conferences (Buckholdt, 1983).

Finally, staff must honor in a timely manner the agreements made to family members. Lack of follow-through can create mistrust and insecurity, which exacerbate existing problems. Following-through on agreements communicates to the family member "The staff values you enough to keep their word; you are an important person to us," it builds trust for future encounters, and helps the resident and family member view staff as being on their side rather than as adversaries, as in the following example (Kelley, 1997):

> The fact that they put credence to what I tell them, like if I suggest something and they follow through, that makes me feel really good.

Finally, as staff follow through on agreed-on goals, they should keep looking for alternatives to resolve the conflict if the original plan does not work.

FAMILY INVOLVEMENT IN CARE INTERVENTION: A FAMILY–STAFF PARTNERSHIP

One program that can defuse conflict between families and staff and that maximizes effective family involvement in care is the family–staff partnership intervention, the Family Involvement in Care (FIC) protocol (Maas et al., 1994). Satisfaction is likely to increase among all parties involved—staff, family, and residents—when the family members and staff act as partners rather than opponents. When the partnership has clearly outlined and agreed on roles for family and staff, these partners are able to work in ways that complement each other. The FIC intervention is a step-by-step method designed to help DSCU staff and family members work together to provide the best care for the resident (Maas et al., 1994; Maas & Swanson, 1991). The main feature of the FIC intervention is the family–staff caregiving partnership, which emphasizes cooperation between staff and families and includes specific and clearly outlined roles for family caregivers (Duncan & Morgan, 1994). The family member's role is "negotiated," or decided on, through a four-step process. The goals of the FIC intervention are to (Maas et al., 1994)

- Decrease staff and family stress
- Decrease dissatisfaction with caregiving roles for both staff and family
- Improve the quality of the relationships among staff, families, and residents
- Increase job satisfaction levels of staff members
- Improve staff attitudes about families
- Maximize the cognitive and functional abilities of residents and reduce their inappropriate behaviors

This complementary and cooperative approach has several benefits: It enhances the quality of care for residents, creates an opportunity for families to provide both relief and assistance to staff, allows DSCU staff to educate family members about their loved ones' problems, brings family and staff together as plans are made for residents' care, and promotes a more satisfying level of involvement for families in the care of their loved ones.

The FIC intervention protocol is composed of four key elements, described in more detail in the following sections (Maas et al., 1994; Maas & Swanson, 1991).

ORIENTATION OF THE FAMILY TO THE FACILITY AND THE PROPOSED PARTNERSHIP ROLE

The first step of the FIC intervention is to orient family members to both the facility and the idea of becoming a partner with the staff. After admission, the primary nurse assigned to the family and resident contacts the family caregiver and orients him or her to the facility. For example, the nurse may take the family members on a tour of the facility, offering explanations about services, activities, or opportunities for privacy; review with family members the facility's philosophies and policies, helping family members to better understand the "why" behind the "what" of activities; and introduce family members to various staff members— dietary, housekeeping, nurses and nursing assistants, secretaries—offering explanations of their roles and responsibilities.

The second step is for the primary nurse to introduce the idea that one of the philosophies of the facility is to develop a partnership between families and staff in caring for the loved one with dementia. The nurse then orients family members to this idea: How the family and staff can become partners in caring for the resident is explained and that family members are encouraged to discuss and ask questions. Designation of one member to assume a leadership role (i.e., representing other family members) in the partnership by participating in the partnership contract is made. The family representative is asked to review and sign the Family and Staff Statement of Partnership Intent, an agreement that both the family member and the staff will work to develop their partnership. Finally, a time for staff to meet with the family representative to work out the specifics of their partnership agreement is set.

NEGOTIATION AND FORMATION OF THE FAMILY–STAFF PARTNERSHIP CONTRACT

At the next meeting, the primary nurse and family representative discuss the goals of the care that will be provided to the resident, including the nursing interventions that will be used to reach these goals. Family representatives are expected and encouraged to contribute to the discussion, to offer their thoughts, feelings, and suggestions. This discussion may include the anticipated routine or methods of managing the resident's care (e.g., bath time, medication administration schedule, physical or occupational therapy routines, psychosocial therapies or groups, adult day services); the family representative's preferences for the resident's attire, possessions, name by which he or she will be addressed, activities, food, and daily routine; and family insights about care strategies or routines that have been successful. During the discussion, the family representative and the primary nurse decide on the goals and approaches to be implemented, which are then put in writing. One copy is given to the family member and one is placed in the resident's chart, becoming the basis of the nursing care plan.

After the goals and approaches are outlined, the staff and family negotiate the Family–Staff Partnership Contract. This contract delineates the type and extent of the family's involvement in the care of the resident. Family members choose activities in which they want to be involved, including the number of activities and their specific involvement in each activity (e.g., how often, how long, how much). At the same time, expectations for staff involvement (Schwartz & Vogel, 1990) and/or assistance are discussed and agreed on (e.g., "The resident will be bathed and dressed by 9 A.M., when a family member arrives for an outing"). These specifics are written down and become the contract or formal agreement between the family and the facility staff. Like the care plan, copies of the Family–Staff Partnership Contract are given to the family representative and placed in the resident's chart.

EDUCATION OF FAMILY MEMBERS FOR INVOLVEMENT IN CARE

The third step of the FIC intervention involves the education, both formal (e.g., resident and family teaching) and informal (e.g., information sharing as part of conversation and communication), of family members. Family members' education begins with their first contact with the primary nurse, their orientation to the facility, and their introduction to the partnership-in-care ideas. Ongoing education and information sharing provides family members with tools that help them

cope with the resident and manage their own feelings, and increases their understanding of residents' behavior and methods in order to promote optimal functioning. Information and understanding of the care plan enhances the family
members' sense of control and increases the likelihood of family–staff cooperation
in the care plan (Rubin & Shuttlesworth, 1983).

Specific educational foci and strategies used are outlined in the following
list. With each of the foci and strategies, the nurse provides information about the
rationale for resident behavior and the interventions used. Likewise, opportunities for families to ask questions, discuss concerns, and become involved in the
process of resident care are always part of the educational intervention (Maas et
al., 1994; Smith et al., 1993).

- A "Welcome!" brochure, which explains both general beliefs about care and
  the partnership concept, is presented to each family member during their first
  contact with the primary nurse. The nurse uses the brochure as a tool to
  explain general principles of care that are used in the facility and that are recommended for families. Likewise, the description of the partnership provides
  a simple outline of ways the facility hopes to involve the family in the care of
  the resident.
- Written information about the resident's particular cognitive, physical, and/or
  mental health problem is provided to the family representative to increase
  understanding of the resident's behavior and the rationale for the care strategies that are used.
- A manual that specifically describes personal care strategies, therapeutic
  activities, and psychosocial rehabilitation modalities (including both illustra-
  tions and examples) is presented to the family representative and the staff.
- The nurse provides general information about care and specific ideas to make
  the family member's involvement in the resident's personal care more meaningful and enjoyable for both.
- Family members are informed about therapeutic activities that may be beneficial to the resident (e.g., music, reminiscence, validation, remotivation, sensory retraining) and about ways to use these methods on a one-to-one basis
  during visits or activities, or while care is being provided.
- Family members are encouraged to assume a specific role in the psychosocial
  rehabilitation of residents, such as co-leading therapeutic groups with staff,
  using one of the methods noted above.

FOLLOW-UP EVALUATION AND
RENEGOTIATION OF THE PARTNERSHIP CONTRACT

The fourth and final step in the FIC intervention is to schedule regular meetings
that allow the family representative and the primary nurse to discuss the resident's
care and the status of their partnership to date, including the evaluation of goals

and approaches in use, discussion of the resident's status and the family member's satisfaction with his or her level of involvement, and renegotiation of the family–staff contract. The most important aspect to keep in mind during these regular meetings is to ensure ongoing communication and evaluation. Two strategies are used to accomplish this goal: monthly meetings, either by telephone or in person (i.e., if the family is unable to meet face-to-face, the nurse contacts the family member by telephone), that involve the primary nurse and family representative, and quarterly care planning meetings that include the primary nurse, other staff members involved in the resident's care, the family representative, other interested family members, and even the resident, if appropriate. The primary nurse is the facilitator of the discussion, encouraging family/staff contributions and solving problems, and helping the group to maintain focus. At these quarterly meetings, family members share with the staff their memories of the residents and their lives prior to admission; family members bring memorabilia and other items from home that are reminiscent of the person's past and may be used in therapeutic modalities; staff share their observations/experiences with the resident and family members; care strategies are reviewed by the family members and staff and revisions to the care plan are adopted by mutual decision; the family–staff contract is renegotiated, including the activities and the specific level of family involvement in each; and copies of the care plan and the family–staff contract are provided to the family representative and placed in the resident's chart.

SUMMARY

Traditional outsider–insider role relationships of family members and staff that develop when people with dementia transition to a nursing facility are not optimal relationships for family members, staff, or residents. Rather, family members and staff should view themselves as partners in care from the beginning of their relationships. The FIC intervention provides a four-step model to guide DSCU staff as they seek to establish and maintain partnerships with family members (Spencer, 1991). This partnership model creates a legitimate role for family members to play when placement diminishes it and increases the sense of control and satisfaction among family members by involving them in decisions, sharing information, encouraging their involvement, and permitting them to participate as fully as desired in their loved ones' care. The FIC provides both relief and assistance to staff by reducing staff–family conflicts and providing assistance with care. This cooperative model has the potential to benefit all parties involved (Maas et al., 1994).

CONCLUSION

Placement in a nursing facility can be a difficult adjustment for the resident and family members. Often, the move to long-term care causes a dramatic change in the role of the family member from primary caregiver to "visitor" (Maas et al., 1994). Some family caregivers feel that they have little control over and little input in the resident's care. They are asked to allow strangers to provide the care that they have given in the past. In many cases, family members may feel relief because they no longer carry the burden of having to provide daily care. However, the lack of control over and involvement in their loved ones' care can create both stress and dissatisfaction with the care provided by the nursing facility staff (Duncan & Morgan, 1994; Maas et al., 1994). This problem is complicated further by attitudes and beliefs that may be maintained by staff. Too often, staff view family visits and requests as unnecessary obstacles or hindrances to their work. Some staff members may even resent family members' participation in the care of "their" resident (Clifford, 1985). Furthermore, family members may find it difficult to maintain satisfying relationships with the person with dementia because of the changes the disease evokes, unclear and often uneasy family–staff relationships, outright conflict with staff, and other structural or organizational barriers that are a part of institutional living (e.g., lack of privacy, problems with roommates, no telephones in rooms, facility policies or procedures) (Buckwalter & Hall, 1987).

Staff should give much consideration to the kinds of stress that family members may be experiencing, including long-standing stresses within the family, stress that is part of their life outside of caring for their loved ones, and stress that was or is part of their loved ones' living in a nursing facility. Anything that staff can do to prevent problems by defusing situations before they reach crisis proportions will help family members, residents, and themselves to be more comfortable. To achieve this goal, the following problem-solving steps should be kept in mind: Accept the family member's concern as real, get all of the facts, decide on a plan of action, and evaluate and follow through (Smith et al., 1993).

Family members can be an important resource for providing good-quality care if staff can "tune in" to their feelings and concerns, help them understand what is being done and why, and let them know that the staff do understand and care (Rubin & Shuttlesworth, 1983).

REFERENCES

Bowers, B.J. (1988). Family perceptions of care in a nursing home. *Gerontologist, 28,* 361–368.

Brody, E.M. (1985). Parent care as a normative stress. *Gerontologist, 25*(1), 19–29.

Buckholdt, D.R. (1983). The family conference: The social control of human development. *Journal of Family Issues, 4*(4), 613–632.

Buckwalter, K.C., & Hall, G.R. (1987). Families of the institutionalized older adult: A neglected resource. In T.H. Brubaker (Ed.), *Aging, health and family* (pp. 176–196). Newbury Park, CA: Sage Publications.

Clifford, A. (1985). Your mother is ours now. *Journal of Gerontological Nursing, 10*(9), 44.

Duncan, M.T., & Morgan, D.L. (1994). Sharing the caring: Family caregivers' views of their relationships with nursing home staff. *Gerontologist, 34*(2), 235–244.

George, L., & Gwyther, L. (1986). Caregiver well-being: A multidimensional examination of family caregivers of demented adults. *Gerontologist, 26*(3), 253–259.

Kelley, L. (1997). *Family perceptions of evaluation of care in dementia special care units.* Unpublished manuscript, University of Iowa College of Nursing, Iowa City.

Maas, M., Buckwalter, K.C., Kelley, L., & Stolley, J.M. (1991). Family members' perceptions: How they view care of Alzheimer's patients in a nursing home. *Journal of Long-Term Care Administration, 19*(1), 21–25.

Maas, M., Buckwalter, K.C., Swanson, E., Specht, J., Tripp-Reimer, T., & Hardy, M. (1994). The caring partnership: Staff and families of persons institutionalized with Alzheimer's disease. *American Journal of Alzheimer's Care and Related Disorders and Research, 9*(6), 21–30.

Maas, M., & Swanson, E. (1991). Family Involvement in Care. Grant funded in part by the National Center for Nursing Research.

Max, W., Webber, P., & Fox, P. (1995). Alzheimer's disease: The unpaid burden of caring. *Journal of Aging and Health, 7*, 179–199.

Morris, J., & Murphy, K. (1995, November). *The role of the family in special care: A family partnership program.* Paper presented at the Gerontological Society of America 50th Annual Scientific Meeting, Los Angeles.

Rubin, A., & Shuttlesworth, G.E. (1983). Engaging families as a support resource in nursing home care: Ambiguity in the subdivision of tasks. *Gerontologist, 23*, 632–636.

Schwartz, A.N., & Vogel, M.E. (1990). Nursing home staff and residents' families role expectations. *Gerontologist, 30*(1), 49–53.

Smith, M., Buckwalter, K.C., & Mitchell, S. (1993). *Friend or foe? Families of the institutionalized older adult. Geriatric Mental Health Training Series.* Cedar Rapids, IA: Abbe, Inc.

Spencer, B. (1991). Partners in care: The role of families in dementia care units. In D.H. Coons (Ed.), *Specialized dementia care units* (pp. 189–204). Baltimore: The Johns Hopkins University Press.

Stephens, M., Kinney, J., & Ogrocki, P. (1991). Stressors and well-being among caregivers to older adults with dementia: The in-home versus nursing home experience. *Gerontologist, 31*, 217–223.

Wilson, H. (1989). Family caregiving for a relative with Alzheimer's dementia: Coping with negative choices. *Nursing Research, 38*(2), 94–98.

Zarit, S.H., & Whitlatch, C.J. (1992). Institutional placement: Phases of the transition. *Gerontologist, 32*, 665–672.

III

Management Strategies

8

Environment—
A Silent Partner in Caregiving

Elizabeth C. Brawley, I.I.D.A., I.F.D.A.

Environmental approaches are not appreciated, even though they often have a faster, safer, and more effective impact than other interventions. While Alzheimer's disease can be neither prevented nor arrested, environmental options offer some of the best conditions to maximize quality of life during the course of this tragic disorder.

Gene D. Cohen, M.D., Ph.D. (1996)

Aging is a process, not an illness. Although steps can be taken to reduce the probability of diseases, the process of aging persists. Vision and hearing loss; reduced stamina, strength, agility, and range of motion; slowed mental processing; and sleep disorders are factors in the aging process. Many changes that result from aging, such as the following, have a direct impact on behavior:

Sensory deficits (e.g., vision, hearing)

Increased response time

Decreased ability to adjust to new environments

Increased sensitivity to medications

Shift in the center of gravity

Flexion at the hips and knees

Decreased righting responses

Decreased proprioception (i.e., reception of stimuli produced by the organism)

Stiffer, shuffling gait

Increasing frailty can make it difficult, if not dangerous, for an older person to climb stairs, bathe, or cook. In addition, the presence of glare, noise, and odors in the environment is particularly aggravating and affects comfort levels significantly (Brawley, 1997). Floor and wall surfaces, as well as furniture, should have low-sheen or matte finishes that diminish reflected light within the environment. The goal of adaptation is to help people live comfortably. Without question, many adaptations and adaptive devices can eliminate hazards and make independent living easier. Addressing the needs of residents of nursing facilities who experience cognitive impairment with good seating, improved lighting, shortened walking distances, and access to safe and stimulating outdoor spaces should make the environment more suitable.

People with Alzheimer's disease have special needs. Although many older adults remain physically intact well into the course of Alzheimer's disease, their memories, judgment, and ability to reason are jeopardized. These individuals need increasing levels of care in order to perform the most basic activities of daily living (ADLs) and to prevent harm to themselves. In addition, appropriate therapeutic programs can help support their remaining functional abilities and prevent excess disabilities (Brawley, 1997). However, older adults have varying degrees of ability: Some 90-year-olds feel vigorous and sharp, whereas some 65-year-olds have Parkinson's or Alzheimer's disease and require daily care. Thus, individual needs must be accommodated without relying on a single solution.

In the creation of living environments for people with Alzheimer's disease, facility policy and design criteria can make the difference between a limiting or a healing environment. The residents, their needs, and their activity programs should provide a foundation on which the design is created and define how the building will appear and function. Although the environment cannot ameliorate the behavior problems caused by Alzheimer's disease, it can minimize the fear engendered by what seems to them to be threatening surroundings (Brawley, 1997).

Poor design choices (e.g., inadequate lighting, flooring that produces glare, seating that is too soft or too low to exit safely) are costly in human as well as monetary terms. Design for long-term care settings must be crafted around a program of spatial needs, followed by site planning, and completed by shaping and connecting the necessary spaces, while remaining sensitive to proportion, scale, light, color, and furnishings. It is crucial that spaces and sequences of space reflect the needs of residents. As people become increasingly dependent on their environment to compensate for frailty and sensory losses, it is clear that design is not just an incidental concern but integral to a well-balanced approach (Brawley, 1992). A well-designed environment addresses the chronic conditions of older adults: More than 50% of older people are affected by arthritis, followed by hypertension, hearing impairments (affecting more than 36% of older adults), heart disease, and cataracts and other visual impairments (U.S. Senate Special Committee on Aging, 1991). Well-designed environments help older adults maintain good-quality physical, cognitive, and social functioning, and promote health and safety. In order to achieve these goals, the design of long-term care settings must depart from traditional design models.

PHYSICAL ENVIRONMENT

Environments that support people as they age, promote wellness, and eliminate the possibility of accidents should be understood to be good preventive strategies. Achieving such environments must be given priority by all long-term care facilities, retirement villages, and senior housing developments.

FALLS AND SUPPORTIVE ENVIRONMENTS

In 1987 it was reported that more than 200,000 older adults fracture their hips in falls each year, resulting in death for more than one third and direct care costs in excess of $7 billion (Brozan, 1988). In 1995 the number of older adults experiencing falls increased to 280,000 a year (Petit, 1995). Preventing falls demands the identification of risk factors and a decrease in as many of these risk factors as possible. In his keynote address to the American Hospital Association conference in 1992, former Surgeon General C. Everett Koop stated that "in order to control health care costs, the one thing that we cannot have too much of is prevention" (Koop, 1992). Greater care must be exercised by nursing facility personnel and older people in providing safe outdoor spaces and avoiding interior environmental risks such as loose rugs, inadequate lighting, and hard floors (Petit, 1995).

Environmental hazards, such as the following, should be guarded against in older adults' residences:

Lighting: dark, too dim, glare, shadows

Walking surfaces: uneven, cracked, wet/slippery, or patterned floors

Stairs: edges not clearly defined, poor step design, inadequate handrails

Furniture: too low, too soft, too deep, unstable (e.g., tips easily, on wheels)

Bathroom: slippery tub or shower, lack of handrails, poorly positioned supports

Furnishings/equipment: improper (i.e., unsafe or improperly specified—does not meet residents' needs in the best possible way) furnishings, worn out or broken

Clothing: too long, too loose, flowing

Shoes/slippers: improper fit, too loose, soles are too slick, heels are badly worn

The changes associated with normal aging, as well as the pathologies common to older people, also increase the risk of falls. The risk is at least twice as high in women as it is in men. Not only is there a greater percentage of older women than older men but older women tend to have more brittle bones and may fall more heavily on their hips (Petit, 1995). The probability of falling increases rapidly after age 85, an age group that is growing six times faster than the rest of the population and is the average age of nursing facility residents.

Because many residents are deficient in vitamin D, falls occur more commonly in nursing facilities than they do in people in the same age group living elsewhere in the community (Tinetti & Speechley, 1989). To reduce the incidence of hip fractures and to strengthen bones, particularly women's bones because they are more susceptible to osteoporosis than are men, it may be critical to introduce diets that have a high calcium content. The method used most often is to include dairy products in the diet. However, many older adults dislike milk or are lactose intolerant. An alternative is controlled exposure to sunlight; most of the vitamin D the human body requires is made in the skin under the influence of sunlight. In fact, approximately 10 minutes of summer sun shining on the hands and face is enough to produce 400 International Units of vitamin D, which is twice the recommended dietary allowance for most adults. Whether the body synthesizes it or obtains it from the diet, vitamin D is converted in the body into a hormone with many essential functions, including the regulation of calcium absorption and the maintenance of strong bones (Weininger, 1994).

Environmental interventions can be implemented to prevent or reduce the incidence of falls. For example, contrasting edge strips define stairs clearly and assist with orientation. Well-lit stairways (e.g., about 30 lux or 30 foot-candles) improve safety. Lighting should be arranged to accentuate stairs and avoid or reduce glare. Handrails should be finished in a contrasting accent color.

MOBILITY AND SUPPORTIVE ENVIRONMENTS

After a fall, the fear of a recurrence can drastically limit an individual's mobility; he or she may become more tentative or withdraw. However, erring on the side of overprotection creates a new set of problems related to restricted mobility. It is, therefore, critical that care providers improve their skills in assessing the risks and causes of falls in order to prevent them.

The caregiver's objective is to maintain the ability of older people to function at the highest level that is possible for them. Well-designed lighting; proper flooring materials; level, interesting walkways; and handrails designed for support help to increase mobility for residents. Exercise/mobility increases physical strength and encourages emotional well-being. Environmental factors that directly affect mobility and an adequate amount of exercise are as follows (Brawley, 1997):

1. Lighting—Insufficient lighting and an overabundance of glare are one of the most critical problems in residential settings. Older residents with dementia

need high general illumination levels and consistent light sources in order to eliminate shadows, which may frighten them. When light is insufficient for older people to see well, they tend to give up on activities, even walking.

2. Long Distances—Long corridors are incongruous with the needs of frail residents, whose placement in a long-term care setting may be due to poor ambulation. Dining areas often are located at inconvenient distances from residents' rooms, whereas they are conveniently located for dining room staff and for marketing the facility to the media and potential residents.

3. Wall/Floor Contrast—Because depth perception is impaired in many older people, particularly people with dementia, a sharp contrast between the color/value of the floor and the color/value of the wall is necessary to provide a clear distinction between the vertical wall plane and the horizontal floor plane. This distinction of contrast is an essential element in maintaining balance. Also, it is important to match the vinyl or wood base molding to the wall, not to the floor in order to provide clear definition of where the horizontal floor plane meets the vertical wall surface (Figure 1).

4. Flooring—Carpet can add warmth and a homelike ambiance, provide excellent acoustical value, and reduce glare. It provides a safer walking environment and a much softer surface, should a fall occur. Floor patterns are a concern for older adults in general, many of whom are affected by depth perception problems, and a profound concern for individuals with cognitive impairment. Some patterns may appear to the person with dementia to move, which disturbs balance or otherwise may be confusing. The unsettling effects of feeling unbalanced, coupled with the fear of falling, may forestall older people from continuing to be mobile.

5. Seating—Much of the upholstered furniture used by older adults is too low, too soft, and too deep, putting them at risk for a fall each time they attempt to exit the seat.

6. Handrails—A well-designed handrail provides necessary support for older adults; the oval shape with a broader, flat surface on top can be used for arm support. The broader handrail with a bullnosed-edge detail allows individuals, even those with arthritis, to grasp and then glide along the handrail (see Figure 1).

LIGHT DEPRIVATION AND SUPPORTIVE ENVIRONMENTS

Sleep disorders, depression, and reduced calcium absorption are common problems experienced by older adults who are light deprived. Sleep is controlled by both voluntary (e.g., amount of caffeine intake) and involuntary (i.e., biological) factors. The involuntary factor is the circadian rhythm (i.e., rhythms of the body cycling on a 24-hour "clock" [Singer & Hughes, 1995]) for sleepiness, timed by the circadian pacemaker. Circadian rhythm affects hormonal systems and sets body rhythms, which regulate a host of interrelated biological processes, including body temperature, heart rate, blood pressure, and the sleep–wake cycle, run-

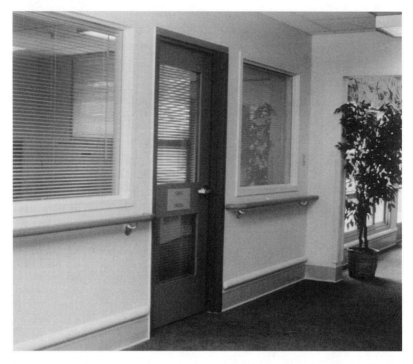

Figure 1.   A hallway in the On-Lok Senior Health Services facility illustrates well the appropriate wall/floor contrast with the cove base matched to the wall color for clear definition. Carpeting absorbs noise and provides a safe walking environment and a soft floor surface in case of falls. A handrail with a broad, flat surface and bullnosed-edge detail provides support. (Photograph courtesy of On-Lok Senior Health Services, San Francisco, California.)

ning approximately 24 hours. Circadian rhythms trigger many daily activities (e.g., hunger/eating, sleeping/awakening), all of which occur at about the same time every day. In addition, "the impairment of circadian rhythms that is characteristic of Alzheimer's disease is also related to agitation" (see Chapter 3).

Daily exposure to bright light and secretion of the hormone melatonin by the pineal gland set the circadian pacemaker and control an individual's level of alertness. Blood levels of circulating melatonin are up to 10 times higher in the body at night than in the day and thus signal the body when it is time to sleep, but as people age, melatonin is produced at night in decreasing amounts. With less circulating melatonin to provide internal stability, it is conceivable that older people are even more dependent on daily light exposure. Older adults, especially those with dementia, may receive levels of light exposure that are insufficient to provide the optimum circadian rhythm.

Older adults tend to become sleepy early in the evening and experience middle-of-the-night awakenings. Many older people exhibit mild symptoms of chronic insomnia. Exposure to bright natural light during the day or to specially designed bright light during the evening has proved effective in improving the quality of older adults' sleep (Campbell et al., 1993). Although interior lighting systems do not adequately synchronize circadian rhythm, daylight is bright enough to be a strong synchronizer (Van Someren et al., 1993); it is freely available, unrestricted, and can be incorporated in building interiors (Campbell et al., 1987).

SEATING

The importance of selecting the proper seating for older people cannot be overemphasized. Typically, older adults sit for extended periods of time, have poor blood circulation, and have difficulty getting into and out of their seats. If more well-designed chairs were available, some residents' mobility would increase. For example, chair arms that extend beyond the chair seat provide more stability for the older person who might otherwise lose balance by propelling forward when exiting the chair. Available space beneath a chair is also necessary to allow a person to place one foot slightly behind the other for balance when rising.

Chairs for older adult users must be superior in quality and comfort: In general, people breathe more easily when standing or sitting erect; chairs that provide lower back support are essential. Well-designed, well-made chairs can be difficult to find, and not all chairs are appropriate for all uses—rocking chairs, dining chairs, lounge chairs, game table chairs, and wingback chairs all have different functions (Figures 2 and 3).

The selection of appropriate dining chairs requires additional consideration. Stability is crucial. Chair arms are essential to support an individual while sitting and rising; they must pass under the table easily. Chairs must be lightweight and sturdy in order to glide well, as casters present an unnecessary hazard. Often, the back of a chair is used as a supportive device, much like a handrail, by frail older adults.

SOCIAL ENVIRONMENT

Many older adults live in unsympathetic, unresponsive social settings, and their feelings of alienation are deepened by the physical conditions of the setting. To be successful, their environment should be configured to maximize their remaining abilities by addressing age-related functional changes. Architects, planners, and designers must challenge the traditional forms and inspire new models in circulation, spatial design, color, and lighting. The clinical model of design, which is based on acute care or hospital design, does not anticipate the requirements of older adults or satisfy the needs of residents of long-term care facilities. The stereotypical image of an immobilized, confined, and isolated resident must be replaced in dementia-specific care settings with one that nurtures physical, social,

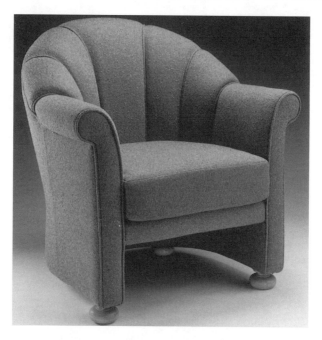

Figure 2.   This upholstered chair demonstrates appropriate, stable design and con-struction. The arms assist the older person in rising and exiting the chair, and there is an adequate amount of space beneath the chair for safety in rising. This chair features a higher-than-normal seat height, which is appropriate for older people, particularly those who are frail. (Photograph courtesy of the Center of Design for an Aging Society, Portland, Oregon. Designer: Eunice Noell. Manufacturer: Senior Style, Ltd. Style: Manhattan.)

and creative activities. The arts are beneficial agents for sustaining health and blunting the effects of Alzheimer's disease: Creative activity programs that include music and dance encourage movement, exercise, and socialization. Painting and sculpture provide outlets for emotional expression, helping to diminish agitation and increase self-esteem.

The design of the hospitable health care setting must recognize "two great human needs, our need for privacy and our need for membership" or inclusion (Davis & Bush-Brown, 1994). Rather than moving residents to central services, it is usually beneficial to deliver decentralized services to groups of residents in clus-tered areas. The growing trend toward small cluster environments, which serve 8–12 people, is an approach through which residents' rooms are located adjacent to central living, dining, and multiple-activity spaces. This design not only elim-inates long corridors but also offers living and dining areas that are residential in scale, creating a homelike atmosphere. With a variety of smaller activity spaces,

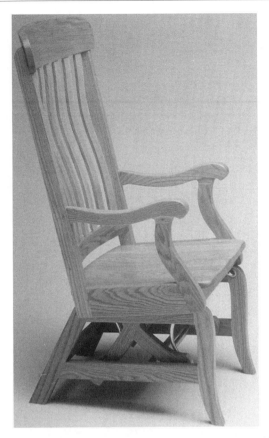

Figure 3.   This oak rocking chair demonstrates appropriate, stable design and construction. The arms assist the older person in rising and exiting the chair, and there is an adequate amount of space beneath the chair for safety in rising. This stable-base rocking chair offers good lower back support. (Photograph courtesy of ADDEN Furniture, Lowell, Massachusetts.)

social gatherings become intimate and can give residents the feeling of having an extended family. Also, residents may feel more secure knowing that they are not far from their rooms. Without the confusion of long corridors, residents are able to see their bedroom door from the living room, dining room, or activity areas. Where multiple corridors exist, strategies should be developed to assist residents, visitors, and staff in order to easily distinguish one area from another. Providing each area with a name similar to that of a street or neighborhood and reinforcing it with visual imagery helps to identify a location. Rather than relying on traditional signage, staff should be creative; they should use identifying memorabilia outside a resident's room that acts as a cueing device (Figure 4). The aroma of cof-

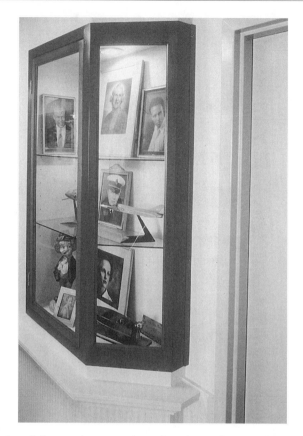

Figure 4.   A well-designed memory box placed outside a resident's room helps to cue residents with memory loss to the correct location of their rooms. (Photograph courtesy of the Irwin Architectural Group, Huntington Beach, California. Architect: Douglas Pancake. The facility pictured is Southwoods Lodge at Hillcrest Retirement Community, La Verne, California.)

fee or the view of a kitchen table and chairs is a more successful cue than arrows or a sign.

A sense of inclusion also can be nurtured by sequences of common or public spaces, carefully joined to walkways. The circulation patterns should reduce conventional arrangements of corridors, elevators, and stairs and introduce dedicated paths, atria, and gardens. Encouraging social activities is effective when residents feel that they are members of a caring community. It nurtures friendships for lonely people, encourages opportunities to feel useful, and above all, stimulates purposeful engagement within a community setting (Davis & Bush-Brown, 1994).

SENSORY ENVIRONMENT

A large body of experimental and clinical data in animals and humans substanti-ates the connection between sensory stimulation and biological responses. The brain and nervous systems directly influence the body's ability to protect itself against illness, as well as to heal itself. The major environmental factors linked, positively or negatively, to physical and emotional health are color, acoustics, aroma, touch and texture, and, especially, lighting.

COLOR

Color strongly influences a person's emotions and his or her entire physiology. Monotonous surroundings may provoke anxiety, fear, and distress. The color red tends to stimulate the nervous system, increasing brain wave activity and sending more blood to the muscles, which accelerates heart rate, blood pressure, and res-piration; the color blue has a tranquilizing effect. Color also affects perception. Thermal comfort can be altered in rooms by using cool tones (e.g., blues, greens) to make people feel cooler and warm tones (e.g., reds, pinks, yellows) to make people feel warmer, although the actual temperature remains the same. Color perception can be affected by texture, placement (i.e., colors adjacent to one another), light sources, reflectance of surrounding surfaces, and aging (e.g., the ability to see variations in hue decreases as a person ages). Choosing color palettes for settings inhabited by older adults requires a great deal of knowledge, skill, and patience. Color choices should reflect the type of activity conducted in the envi-ronment and be selected simultaneously with lighting.

Perhaps the most common error made in selecting colors for environmental settings for older adults with and without cognitive impairment is allowing per-sonal preference to influence choices, rather than choosing what is in the best interest of the resident. Questions that should be asked include is the color selec-tion easily discernible? Are the color values appropriate? Is the contrast strong enough? All people have their own color preferences, and the current color trends can be seductive, but colors must be viewed through the eyes of the person who will live in the environment.

ACOUSTICS

An acoustically comfortable environment is a necessity for older residents. Noise can induce psychological changes that lead to high blood pressure, heart disease, and ulcers, and has been proved to adversely affect visual perception and dimin-ish learning capacity (Welch & Welch, 1970): Literally, it can become too noisy to think. Auditory trauma also incites anger and irritability (Noell, 1994). Acoustics can be improved by selecting interior surfaces and furnishings that do not reflect or amplify sound waves; for example, carpeting muffles the sound of footsteps and serving carts. In addition to prevention, sound absorption can be accomplished through a variety of interventions such as replacing voice-activated paging and public address systems with electronic pagers. Irregularly recessed walls and ceilings provide increased quiet; fabric, wood, acoustic tile, and sound panels may also absorb sound.

AROMAS

Scent has been called *the silent persuader*, influencing mind, body, and health. Smell impulses travel a faster, more direct route to the brain than do visual or auditory impulses, going straight to the limbic system, the emotional center in the brain. Unpleasant smells, such as ammonia, tend to elevate breathing and heart rates. Conversely, pleasant smells, such as spiced apple and light floral scents, tend to reduce stress (Brawley, 1997). Researchers in the field of aromatherapy are exploring ways to use pleasant odors in environments to increase alertness, decrease aggression, and even stimulate the body's natural defenses against disease.

Older adults are particularly vulnerable to indoor pollutants (Baker, 1995). Synthetic materials and adhesives produce varying levels of toxic fumes that off-gas into the environment. Heat and moisture can increase the off-gassing response. Despite this, toxic products, such as cleaning agents, floor wax, and floor wax stripper, are reintroduced into the environment on a daily basis. To minimize older adults' exposure to toxic fumes, wallcovering, flooring materials, fabrics, and furnishings incorporating particleboard should be researched and selected carefully.

The introduction of live plants can increase the amount and quality of fresh air in the environment. A NASA study demonstrated that a combination of ordinary houseplants can remove toxic pollutants, such as formaldehyde, benzene, and trichloroethylene, from indoor air (*San Francisco Chronicle*, n.d.).

TOUCH AND TEXTURE

The environment conveys many messages, especially to older people with cognitive impairment, who, as the disease progresses, rely increasingly on the sensory environment for information. Air quality and tactile comfort (i.e., what we touch and are touched by) are perceived through the skin, the largest sensory organ, yet touch is the most neglected sense. Tactile comfort also relates to the amount of space surrounding a person. Large, open spaces can be disorienting and make people feel vulnerable. For people with cognitive impairment, space may be an even more important issue than has been realized. With popular building trends that incorporate high ceilings in many of the large group areas, the volume of space is increased. Individuals with cognitive impairment are more likely than people without impairment to feel exposed and vulnerable, and may be reluctant to use these spaces.

In creating special care settings, designers often attempt to fabricate a home-like atmosphere: By varying scales in furniture and using a variety of fabrics, finishes, and interesting surface treatments, the environment is enhanced and seems more like "home." Vinyl furniture and plastic-wrapped sofas and chairs are neither familiar nor friendly. With the improved fabrics available, there are many additional upholstery options; for example, fabrics treated with Crypton, a moisture-resistant finish, come in a variety of colorful patterns. Decorative fabrics designed for cubicle curtains also meet the stringent requirements of life/safety codes and may be laundered at temperatures high enough to satisfy health officials. Because they are easily cleaned, many of these colorful, decorative fabrics are an inexpensive alternative to slipcovers, which can hide plastic-covered seat cushions and can disguise even the ugliest vinyl chair.

LIGHTING

The ability to see and function effectively depends on the quantity and quality of the surrounding illumination. Research indicates that inadequate light affects visual acuity and is a factor associated with many falls in older adults (Weston, 1948). Since the experimental work of Weston (1948) and Guth (1957), it has been recognized that, as compared with the average 20-year-old person, the average 60-year-old person requires two to three times the amount of light in order to achieve equal "visibility" and "visual performance," and that this need increases as people age. A Swedish study found a direct correlation between the quality of light in an older person's residence and his or her quality of life (Sorensen & Brunnstrom, 1995). Appetite, physical condition, social interaction, self-confidence, temperament, and general health showed improvement as a result of increased lighting quality. Daylighting refers to architectural design solutions that gather, direct, and reflect natural light deep into single or multistory buildings. Many long-term care settings have little natural light penetrating inside them (Brawley, 1997). Daylighting is an essential design element because it enhances physical and mental well-being and contributes to energy conservation.

Particular attention should be paid to glare (i.e., resulting from the extreme contrast between daylight and the general lighting within the space, light reflected from a shiny surface such as a highly polished floor). Both glare and flicker (i.e., associated with the old magnetic ballasts for fluoresent light sources) may cause discomfort and disability in older adults. These lighting problems can be especially devastating to people with Alzheimer's disease, triggering confusion and disruptive behavior. At times, older adults are mistakenly thought to be avoiding light when they are actually avoiding glare. Electronic ballasts eliminate perceptible flicker, and proper lighting is a key element in the control of glare and flicker.

LIGHTING DESIGNS FOR LONG-TERM CARE SETTINGS

All lighting in long-term care settings should meet the illumination levels for senior housing recommended by the Illuminating Engineering Society of North America (IESNA) in RP-28: Lighting and the Visual Environment for Senior

Living (IESNA, 1998). This document establishes design criteria for lighting and visual elements within the environment. RP-28 is a resource not only for lighting designers but also for the public and state agencies that rely on the IESNA for guidance in establishing state regulations for senior living. However, no consistency exists in lighting requirements from one state to another, and to compound the problem, the variations are widespread (Brawley et al., 1997).

Visibility of objects within the physical environment can be enhanced by providing distinct value contrast between a specific object and its background, well-defined edges, and contrast in changes from one level to another. Because of the yellowing of the lens of the eye with age, lighting with a color-rendering index above 80 also improves visibility for older adults (Brawley et al., 1997).

Fluorescent lighting provides an energy-efficient source of illumination. However, only electronic ballasts should be used with fluorescent lighting fixtures because people with Alzheimer's disease are particularly sensitive to the flicker of magnetic ballasts (e.g., flicker from poor lighting can trigger seizures in people with epilepsy). Fluorescent lamps should have a color-rendering index of 80 or higher and a color temperature of 3,000° or 3,500° Kelvin. These systems produce higher levels of general illumination, with consistent and even distribution of light on room surfaces, and permit the use of energy-efficient fixtures that can be used for ambient and task lighting without diminishing the quality of the overall plan. Light fixture style is an important consideration, particularly when attempting to maintain a homelike atmosphere. One solution is to provide indirect light from fluorescent fixtures, which are designed to be mounted onto architectural features or built-in cabinets. Another option is to provide indirect/direct light for fluorescent fixtures by mounting them behind a valance.

Excessive differences in lighting levels should be avoided in transition areas between driveways, parking lots, courtyards, building entrances, lobbies, and corridors. Because of the thickening of the lens and the reduced size of the pupil, which are factors in normal aging, the eye of an older person is less elastic and adapts slowly to conditions of high contrast between light and dark (McFarland & Fisher, 1955). Problems may be caused by strong directional light. However, even greater problems exist when transitioning from daylight to low interior lighting as a result of the extreme contrast. During the day, outside light can be 100 to 1,000 times greater than interior light levels, and at night, considerably darker. Upon entering a space with a much lower lighting level, older adults may stop or move to one side until their eyes adapt to excessive lighting changes. A good design provides a transition area for their eyes to have time to adjust. Higher light levels in the entry provide a better transition during the day, and electronic dimmers or step-level switching (i.e., part of the lamp is wired to a separate ballast and circuit, which is controlled by a switch) can be utilized at night.

Strong, directional-down light from fixtures recessed in the ceiling should be avoided. Prismatic, wraparound, fluorescent fixtures and fixtures with parabolic diffusers do a good job in illuminating spaces, but are a source of glare because the brightness of the tubes is visible. Unfortunately, these types of lighting seem to be the fixtures of choice for people who do not understand the effects that aging has on vision (Brawley & Noell, 1996).

Indirect light from electrical and daylight sources can deliver high levels of illumination without creating glare. An indirect lighting system directs light toward the ceiling and upper wall areas, reflecting the light off the surfaces that diffuse it. This system produces an even, consistent light level and eliminates shadows. The most consistent forms of indirect lighting are cove lights on wall or ceiling coffers and pendant, indirect lighting fixtures (Figure 5). Bright daylight must be controlled where it enters the building. Sometimes perforated filters, mesh screens, or the use of exterior architectural features or landscaping provide good solutions. In this respect, dark window tints are not good choices because they give the impression that the weather is gray and gloomy, and this may have an effect on the mood or demeanor of older adults. A combination of residential window treatments should be provided for glare and privacy control. Sheer draperies and privacy draperies on separate tracks allow residents to control natural light (Brawley et al., 1996).

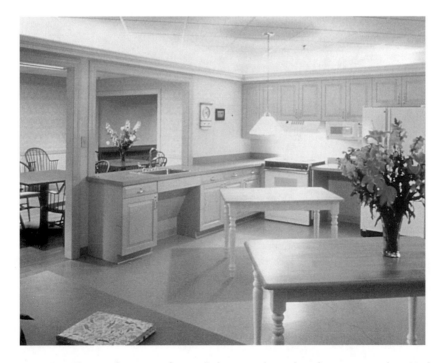

Figure 5.   The combination of cove lighting and pendant fixtures provides excellent lighting sources in hospitals and long-term care facilities. (Photograph courtesy of SMRT Architects, Portland, Maine. Photographer: Robert Darby, AIA. The facility pictured is Sedgewood Commons, Falmouth, Maine.)

Ideally, interior lighting should be provided by windows, atria, skylights, and clerestories. These structures provide a variation in light with the touch of nature, which is important to well-being. Where daylight is not available, lamps (i.e., light tubes) approximating the spectra, or color, of daylight should be used. Effective lighting techniques have the added benefit of conserving energy. All fixtures, with the exception of day use–only activity spaces, should be able to be dimmed or configured for step-level switching to lower the overall lighting evenly. Fluorescent lighting is a good choice for producing a uniform brightness in interior spaces and for raising light levels to balance the daylight on entering a room. In providing higher light levels for older adults, particularly those with Alzheimer's disease, every room or space should be provided with general illumination in addition to specific or task lighting. Natural daylight and dimmable fluorescent light are good indirect light sources for ambient lighting, with daylight often requiring as much planning and control as electrical lighting. The need to balance the light from the windows for visual comfort is important. The following guidelines should be adhered to in order to meet the needs of residents with Alzheimer's disease:

Light levels that are adequate for the visual task

Avoidance of glare (direct and reflected)

Uniformity in general lighting, with areas of interest that are not dramatically different from others

Orientation of lighting to the visual task

Reduction of visual clutter and business

Good color rendition

Locational and directional considerations of light for accident prevention

Balance of daylight and interior ambient light

CONCLUSION

Design solutions that do not meet the needs of older adults, such as the continued use of poor lighting systems, limit their independence and compromise their safety. The burden of consideration must be given to the costs to quality of life rather than simply to the initial design costs.

Design professionals and providers must focus on functional design and integrating gerontological research rather than concentrating only on aesthetics. In believing that design is a catalyst, too much emphasis may be placed on its therapeutic value. The needs of residents and providers are many, diverse, and complex, and they must be addressed in the same fashion. Good design is based on appropriate strategies directed to the special needs of residents, staff, families, and visitors.

Environmental challenges require that designers, architects, and providers rededicate their efforts to supporting comprehensive human values. Promoting independence and dignity in long-term care settings is extremely important, as is the need to provide an atmosphere that considers the individual needs of residents. With a fuller understanding of the unique challenges associated with aging and the challenges posed by Alzheimer's disease and related dementias, architects, facility planners, interior designers, and administrators can better define problems, explore appropriate solutions, and create care environments that actually serve older adults. Developing a philosophy in which the environments created reflect human dignity and vitality benefits health care design professionals and residents alike.

REFERENCES

Baker, B. (1995, September). What ails you? *AARP Bulletin, 36*(8), 2.

Brawley, E.C. (1992, January/February). Alzheimer's disease: Designing the physical environment. *American Journal of Alzheimer's Care and Related Disorders & Research, 7*(1), 3–8.

Brawley, E.C. (1997). *Designing for Alzheimer's disease: Strategies for better care environments.* New York: John Wiley & Sons.

Brawley, E., Dupuy, R., & Noell, E. (1997). *Lighting: Partner in quality care environments.* Paper presented at the Assisted Living Federation Association conference, Phoenix.

Brawley, E., & Noell, E. (1996, July). *The environment: A partner in care.* Paper presented at the Alzheimer's Disease Education Conference, Chicago.

Brozan, N. (1988, December 29). Finally, doctors ask if brutal falls need be a fact of life for the elderly. *The New York Times*, Health Section, p. 17.

Campbell, S.S., Dawson, D., & Anderson, M. (1987). Exposure to light in healthy elderly subjects and Alzheimer's patients. *Physiology and Behavior, 42*, 141–144.

Campbell, S., Dawson, D., & Anderson, M. (1993). Alleviation of sleep maintenance insomnia with timed exposure to bright light. *Journal of the American Geriatrics Society, 41*, 829–836.

Cohen, G.D. (1996, Spring). Treatment of Alzheimer's disease in the absence of cure and prevention. *High Notes.*

Davis, D., & Bush-Brown, A. (1994). *Hospitable design for healthcare and senior communities.* New York: Van Nostrand Reinhold.

Guth, S.K. (1957). Effect of age on visibility. *American Journal of Optometry, American Academy of Optometry, 34*, 463–477.

Illuminating Engineering Society of America. (1998). Recommended practice for lighting and the visual environment for senior living, RP-28. New York: Author.

Koop, C.E. (1992). Keynote address to the American Hospital Association conference, Denver.

McFarland, R.A., & Fisher, D. (1955). Alternation of dark adaptation as a function of age. *Journal of Gerontology, 10*, 424–428.

Noell, E. (1994). *Physiological needs and design responses: Health effects of light and sound.* Paper presented at the annual conference of the American Institute of Architects—Architecture for Health, Washington, DC.

Petit, C. (1995, February 19). Surge in hip fractures feared. *San Francisco Chronicle*, Section B.

San Francisco Chronicle. (n.d.). NASA study. Home & Garden section.

Singer, C., & Hughes, R. (1995, March). Clinical use of bright light in geriatric neuro-psychiatry. *Proceedings of the 3rd International Symposium—Lighting for Aging Vision and Health, Orlando,* pp. 143–146.

Sorensen, S., & Brunnstrom, G. (1995). Quality of light and quality of life: An intervention study among older people. *International Journal of Lighting Research and Technology,* 27(2), 113–119.

Tinetti, M.E., & Speechley, M. (1989). Prevention of falls among the elderly. *New England Journal of Medicine, 320*(16), 1055.

U.S. Senate Special Committee on Aging, American Association of Retired Persons, Federal Council on the Aging, & U.S. Administration on Aging. (1991). *Aging America—Trends and projections* (DHHS Publication No. 91-28001). Washington, DC: Department of Health and Human Services.

Van Someren, E.J.W., Mirmiran, M., & Swaab, D.F. (1993). Non-pharmacological treatment of sleep and wake disturbances in aging and Alzheimer's disease: Chronobiological perspectives. *Behavioral Brain Research, 57,* 235–253.

Weininger, J. (1994, June 15). Sun: Nutrition tips for summer, *San Francisco Chronicle,* Health Section.

Welch, B.L., & Welch, A.S. (Eds.). (1970). *Physiological effects of noise.* New York: Plenum.

Weston, H.C. (1948). *Light, sight, and work.* London: Lewis.

9

Therapeutic Uses of Music to Calm Agitation in Nursing Facility Residents with Dementia

Patricia A. Tabloski, Ph.D., R.N. C.S., and Karen Williams

Mrs. Jones, an 83-year-old woman with Alzheimer's disease, is admitted to a nursing facility after being cared for at home by her daughter for several years. Because of her spatial disorientation and difficulty adjusting to new situations, Mrs. Jones repeatedly tries to leave the facility, saying, "I have to go home to care for my children." The nurses try to redirect her and reassure her, but she becomes increasingly agitated and insistent on leaving. She calls out constantly, refuses to eat, and will not lie down on her bed. Finally, the supervising nurse phones Mrs. Jones's physician to request a calming medication, which can be administered on an as-needed basis. This medication seems to lessen Mrs. Jones's agitation and is used frequently throughout the next week. When Mrs. Jones's daughter visits her mother, she is shocked to find her asleep in her chair at 2:00 P.M. Her daughter is very upset when she learns that a sedating medication has been prescribed, and she states that her mother was never a person who napped or took pills. She demands to know why the nursing facility has been "drugging my mother." The daughter requests that the medication be discontinued immediately and nonpharmacological measures be used in the future to control her mother's agitation. The nurses are not sure how to proceed with the plan of care.

Management of agitated behaviors can be a challenging experience for people providing care to older adults with dementia. About 60% of all nursing facility residents have been diagnosed with probable Alzheimer's disease or some other form of cognitive impairment (Dellasaga & Schellenbarger, 1992). The effects of these cognitive impairments are far reaching and may alter residents' mood and their ability to function independently. One mood disturbance in dementia, agitation, can be particularly troublesome. Cohen-Mansfield and Billig (1986) define agitation as "inappropriate verbal, vocal, or motor activity that is not explained by needs or confusion per se." An agitated resident may yell, pace, scream, bite and kick, and wander either continuously or periodically. Often, these behaviors endanger the resident, caregivers, and other residents, and socially isolate the resident from enjoyable activities. This behavior disorder may begin a vicious cycle in which the resident is isolated in his or her room so as not to disturb others, and, thus, the resident becomes lonely, bored, or both. This cycle results in further agitation, increased demands for attention and care, and increased confusion.

The traditional nursing staff and physician responses to these behaviors were to administer psychotropic medications and physical restraints. The Omnibus Budget Reconciliation Act (OBRA) of 1987 made health care workers aware that interventions other than chemical and physical restraints were needed to help people with cognitive impairment maintain their autonomy, dignity, and quality of life. Common side effects of neuroleptic and psychotropic drugs include gait impairment, increased falling, difficulty swallowing, diminished cognitive function, and paradoxical increases in agitation (Corrigan, 1989; Knopman & Sawyer-Demaris, 1993). Activities of daily living (ADLs), such as mouth care, bathing, application of wound care dressings, and administration of medications, may not be accomplished because of an agitated resident's refusal to cooperate with these procedures. Clearly, the risks of medicating the resident who is agitated are great and the benefits are unpredictable.

Part of the problem caregivers face in providing appropriate interventions for people with cognitive impairment and agitated behaviors is lack of education and training in the manifestations of dementia and ways to manage the resultant behaviors without resorting to chemical or physical restraints. These measures may exacerbate the behavior disorders that are the target of interventions and can contribute to additional difficulties.

ENVIRONMENTAL MODIFICATIONS

The search for appropriate interventions to manage the behavioral manifestations of cognitive impairment have led from chemical and physical restraints to environmental modifications. The Progressively Lowered Stress Threshold (PLST) model was formulated by Hall and Buckwalter (1987) as a response to these behaviors. According to the PLST model, older adults with dementia of the Alzheimer's type experience declining cognitive and functional abilities and increasing difficulty in coping with stress. Because of internal and external demands, their behavior becomes progressively dysfunctional and, frequently, catastrophic as the level of stress increases. The model proposes that if environmental conditions are modified, stress can be reduced, functional adaptive behaviors will be promoted, and people with dementia will exhibit fewer inappropriate behaviors and maintain their cognitive and functional abilities longer.

NOT MUSIC THERAPY BUT MUSIC AS THERAPY

Most professional caregivers are familiar with music as an organized therapy delivered by a music therapist in order to stimulate reminiscence and social interaction. However, few caregivers have used music as an intervention integrated into the regular plan of care as an alternative or a supplement to chemical and physical restraints. Professional caregivers are still novices at thinking beyond the medical model and using their technical knowledge to craft a therapeutic, resident-centered environment. Many caregivers attempt to control or manage residents' behavior rather than try to understand the source of the problem and alter the environment in order to promote maximum potential within the limits of the residents' remaining cognitive abilities. Until caregivers make the transition from a control paradigm to a resident-centered paradigm they cannot provide truly individualized care.

Music is one environmental modification that has been used to reduce agitated behaviors in nursing facility residents with cognitive impairment. Anecdotal evidence relates that music helps to reduce agitated behaviors. Residents who have not been verbal or demonstrative in years suddenly begin singing or smiling when a familiar tune is played. Often, residents who have played instruments continue to play complicated musical pieces perfectly despite severe cognitive impairment, although they cannot name the piece or the composer. In addition to exhibiting decreases in socially unacceptable behaviors, residents who are exposed to music exhibit increases in socially acceptable behaviors. For instance, after listening to calming music, some residents assisted others in wheelchairs, several spoke in softer tones rather than yelled, and some began to move their extremities rhythmically in time to the music (Tabloski, McKinnon-Howe, & Remington, 1995).

Residents need not have been musicians or be categorized as music lovers in order to respond positively to music. Even residents with dementia, who have severe impairment in language ability, orientation, and judgment, may be able to experience and appreciate a music intervention. Studies have documented numerous physiological effects of music. Increased relaxation was evidenced by EEG tracing, which reveals increased alpha brain activity patterns (alpha brain waves indicate deep relaxation or the first stage of sleep; Harvey & Rapp, 1988). Schorr (1993) used calming music to decrease pain perception in women with rheumatoid arthritis. Music played during bronchoscopy reduced discomfort and coughing, and Dubois, Bartter, and Pratter (1995) concluded that music is a simple, inexpensive, and nonpharmacological intervention that increases comfort levels. Casby and Holm (1994) found that both classical music and older-adult favorites (e.g., songs from the World War II and postwar eras) reduced the incidence of repetitive disruptive vocalizations in people with dementia residing in nursing facilities (Norberg, Melin, & Asplund, 1986). Gerdner and Swanson (1993) studied the effects of individualized music on five nursing facility residents with dementia. Music was chosen with assistance from family members, who identified each resident's music preferences and the importance of music in his or her life. Results revealed an overall reduction of agitated behaviors during the music intervention and a further reduction 1 hour postintervention with both types of music.

Goddaer and Abraham (1994) studied the effects of relaxing music used as a way to reduce residents' perceptions of noxious noise in the dining room and to introduce an intentionally relaxing sound source. They postulated that the reduced perception of noxious noise would lessen physiological and psychological responses to the noise, including agitated behaviors. Their results revealed decreases in agitated behaviors from baseline when music was played. Such environmental manipulations may allow facility staff to concentrate time and attention on functional activities instead of on behavior modification or management. Furthermore, the addition of calming music may diminish irritating noise and improve the environment of the nursing facility for residents and staff. Theoretically, a calmer staff should be better able to provide care to difficult, agitated nursing facility residents, who may resist their efforts. Tabloski, McKinnon-Howe, and Remington (1995) examined the use of calming music as a way of decreasing agitated behaviors in nursing facility residents with cognitive impairment. Results revealed significant decreases in agitation scores during the playing of classical music and for a 30-minute period following the intervention. They concluded that music may provide a way for caregivers to decrease agitation by nonpharmacological methods.

STEPS IN A MUSIC INTERVENTION

The steps to take in a music intervention are to assess the resident for agitation and music preferences, choose the music, set up an intervention schedule, and assess the outcome of the intervention.

RESIDENT ASSESSMENT

Before a music intervention can be initiated, residents should be examined carefully for physical or psychological conditions that may cause agitation: They may be hungry, tired, soiled, thirsty, in pain, lonely, or bored. Many times, frail older people with dementia have atypical presentation of disease, with agitation being the first sign of urinary tract infection, bedsores, or fecal impaction. Careful assessment of vital signs, bowel and bladder function, skin condition, and fluid intake is indicated. Once staff establish that a resident is agitated as a result of his or her cognitive impairment, a music intervention can be implemented with confidence. The authors urge careful observation of the resident during the first 5 minutes of the intervention because it is usually within this period of time that initial response can be assessed. If the resident does not demonstrate an initial positive response to the music, it should be discontinued and the resident should be reassessed for secondary causes of agitation such as physical or psychological distress.

Staff also must assess residents' sleep/activity pattern during a 24-hour period. Preliminary observation of agitated residents for whom calming music was played during the day in order to ease their agitation reveals that their sleep patterns may be disrupted, with an increase in nighttime agitation. It is possible that agitation is a way for residents to expel excess energy and that this daytime release of energy may promote more restful sleep at night. Because sleep/rest cycles tend to break down in the later stages of dementia, calming music may promote periods of consolidated sleep, which may improve function in agitated residents. The music intervention should be implemented at night rather than during the day so that further disruption of the sleep/rest cycle is not the unintended result. Clearly, further research is needed to assess this complicated relationship between daytime activity and nighttime sleep in residents with agitation. In the meantime, caregivers are urged to consider using a 24-hour time frame when assessing response to calming music and careful monitoring for changes in sleep patterns.

When assessing agitation in a resident with dementia, it is important to ascertain whether the agitated behaviors he or she manifests are troublesome to the caregivers/dementia-specific care unit (DSCU) or the resident. For instance, a resident who paces and wanders may be working off excess energy and getting much-needed exercise. However, if the resident wanders into another resident's room and attempts to lie down on the bed, it becomes a problem for the DSCU. It is likely that staff, residents, and families will be upset by this activity. The wandering resident requires redirection to safe places to walk and lie down, and a variety of visual barriers can be used to discourage wandering. A large family picture outside the resident's room may help him or her to identify the appropriate room. However, if the wanderer refuses to eat, accept care, or lie down to rest, and develops ankle or foot edema secondary to constant movement, the agitated behavior becomes a problem for the resident and requires assessment and management.

Some questions caregivers may wish to ask in making an assessment follow:

- What is the person looking for?
- Does the person have basic needs that are not being met?
- Can the family provide insight into the behavior?
- How can care be provided to this resident within the framework of his or her wandering behaviors?

- Do the agitated behaviors truly justify treatment, or is staff attempting to control inconvenient behaviors?
- Are environmental conditions contributing to the problem behaviors? Can the environment be adjusted to promote more appropriate function?
- Are physiological factors such as pain, hunger, thirst, or oncoming illness a potential source of agitation? Has staff checked the resident's vital signs, bowel sheet, and skin condition, or sent urine for culture?
- Are psychological factors (e.g., loneliness, boredom, fear) a potential source of agitation? Has staff provided the attention and nurturing the resident needs in order to feel comfortable in the facility?
- Do these behaviors result from medication use? Has staff overused medications in an attempt to control behavior? Has staff provided nonpharmacological interventions along with medication administration? (Although psychotropic drugs may be used, they may exacerbate the behavior disorder and cause a variety of troublesome side effects such as increased confusion, rebound anxiety, and movement disorders.)
- Is staff expecting a "quick fix"? Does staff have all the information necessary?
- What is the resident like at night?
- Who is the person who has been diagnosed with dementia? How can staff best provide resident-centered care?

Music is not an effective intervention for all residents with dementia (e.g., deaf residents or residents with profound hearing impairment). Some residents may respond more positively to visual stimuli (e.g., pictures of family, photographs of tranquil forest scenes) or tactile stimuli (e.g., fabrics such as silk, stuffed animals). This determination must be made before planning a music intervention.

CHOICE OF MUSIC

Once the resident has been assessed, music for the intervention should be chosen. Many different types of music can be used to reduce behavior disorders, and music therapists can assist staff in choosing appropriate recordings. A music history can be obtained from family members before the resident is admitted to the nursing facility so that his or her favorite music is readily available to staff should agitation become a problem during the period of adjustment to the facility. The family may also bring in a recording of the resident's favorite music. This approach provides an individualized response to reducing agitation. Families may state that their loved one played a certain recording on a regular basis or that he or she associates the recording with a pleasant memory (e.g., a wedding, birth of a child or grandchild). It is important that music that is associated with unpleasant events (e.g., death of a loved one) not be chosen. The authors recommend that the recording be at least 15 minutes long in order to hold the attention of the resident with dementia and to achieve a calming effect.

If staff are unsure about which musical selections may benefit the resident, they should try a variety of recordings and note the effect of each. Ethnic music (e.g., polkas, the tango), religious music (e.g., choir, organ), big band tunes, marches or patriotic music, Broadway show tunes, and opera and classical selections all may be appropriate. For example, if classical music is chosen, the recording should have a slow tempo, soft dynamic levels, and repetitive themes (Clair, 1996). In addition to decreasing agitation levels, familiar classical compositions may evoke pleasant memories. Compact discs and audiotapes used for relaxation featuring natural sounds (e.g., birds chirping, water running) are popular. The volume of the music should be set carefully so that the resident can easily hear the music without it being so loud that it blocks conversation or inquiries from caregivers or visitors. Individual headsets or earphones may be used if the resident can tolerate the apparatus and if the music is bothersome to others in the immediate area. Headsets may also be useful when music is played at night or when the resident lives with a roommate who is trying to sleep.

A music library can be developed in the nursing facility in order for staff to have 24-hour access to the selections and to use music when needed for residents who are agitated.

MUSIC INTERVENTION SCHEDULE

Once the caregiver has observed that the resident responds well to music and that he or she demonstrates decreased levels of agitation, the best time of day to initiate a music intervention should be addressed. Additional research is needed to ascertain the optimal time. For residents who sundown, or become agitated in the late afternoon and/or early evening, it may be appropriate to play music 30 minutes before the onset of their peak agitation period. They may be more receptive to calming music before they reach peak agitation levels and, thus, music may prove effective in decreasing problem behaviors; this may be especially true for people who pace or wander. These residents may be too agitated to sit long enough to listen to music. They may attempt to leave the room in which the music is being played and, thus, may not benefit from the intervention.

It is important that music not be played continuously because when it is, it ceases to be an intervention and becomes part of a noisy/disruptive environment that residents tune out. A droning television set, recordings played over the public address system, or radios left on continuously eventually blend into the background and go unnoticed. Music should be used selectively and cautiously in order for it to remain effective and worthy of the attention of residents who are agitated.

ASSESSMENT OF OUTCOMES

The effect of the music on individual residents must be quantified to ensure that the selection of music and timing of the intervention are appropriate. Formal rating scales, such as the Agitated Behavior Scale (Corrigan, Mysiw, Gribble, & Chock, 1992), can be used, but staff may wish to target and quantify one or two of the most troublesome or disruptive behaviors and use one or both as a baseline. For example, one resident's yelling is a problem and proves disruptive to other residents living on the DSCU. Staff should count the number of times per hour the resident yells and note the peak periods during which the yelling occurs. The music deemed appropriate may then be played 1) during the peak periods of yelling for several days, with the effect(s) noted, and 2) 30 minutes before the peak periods of yelling, with the effect(s) noted. Similarly, the music selection can be varied and the effect(s) quantified. In this way, staff will obtain an objective measure of the effect of the music and will feel confident that they are pursuing the appropriate intervention.

CONCLUSION

Caregivers are in desperate need of nonpharmacological interventions that can ease agitation in nursing facility residents with cognitive impairment. Music holds promise as a way to decrease agitation and increase the quality of life for these residents without exposing them to the potentially harmful side effects of psychotropic medications. In addition to decreasing agitation, music may increase socially acceptable, positive behaviors and may evoke pleasant memories and feelings that may help to alleviate agitation (Gerdner & Swanson, 1993). It is probably overly simplistic to ask "Haldol or Haydn?" when attempting to alleviate agitation in residents, but effective, low-cost, nonpharmacological, environmental interventions such as music offer hope. The preliminary data are promising, but further research that documents the calming effect of the type of music selected, the timing of the intervention, and the response to music within a 24-hour time frame is needed.

REFERENCES

Casby, J.A., & Holm, M.B. (1994). The effect of music on repetitive disruptive vocalizations of persons with dementia. *American Journal of Occupational Therapy, 48*(10), 883–889.

Clair, A.A. (1996). *Therapeutic uses of music with older adults.* Baltimore: Health Professions Press.

Cohen-Mansfield, J., & Billig, N. (1986). Agitated behaviors in the elderly: I. A conceptual review. *Journal of the American Geriatrics Society, 34,* 722–727.

Corrigan, J.D. (1989). Development of a scale for assessment of agitation following traumatic brain injury. *Journal of Clinical Experimental Neuropsychology, 1,* 261–277.

Corrigan, J.D., Mysiw, W.J., Gribble, M.W., & Chock, S.K.L. (1992). Agitation, cognition and attention during post-traumatic amnesia. *Brain Injury, 6*(2), 155–160.

Dellasaga, C., & Schellenbarger, T. (1992). Discharge planning for cognitively impaired elderly adults. *Nursing & Health Care, 23*, 526–531.

Dubois, J., Bartter, T., & Pratter, M. (1995). Music improves patient comfort level during outpatient bronchoscopy. *Chest, 108*(1), 129–130.

Gerdner, L.A., & Swanson, E.A. (1993). Effects of individualized music on confused and agitated elderly patients. *Archives of Psychiatric Nursing, 5*, 284–291.

Goddaer, J., & Abraham, L. (1994). Effects of relaxing music on agitation during meals among nursing home residents with severe cognitive impairment. *Archives of Psychiatric Nursing, 8*(3), 150–158.

Hall, G., & Buckwalter, K. (1987). The progressively lowered threshold theory in caring for adults with Alzheimer's disease. *Archives of Psychiatric Nursing, 1*, 399–406.

Harvey, A.W., & Rapp, L. (1988). Music soothes the troubled soul. *AD Nurse,* (3), 19–22.

Knopman, P.S., & Sawyer-Demaris, S. (1993). Practical approach to managing problems in dementia patients. *Geriatrics, 45*, 27–35.

Norberg, A., Melin, E., & Asplund, K. (1986). Reactions to music, touch, and object presentation in the final stage of dementia. An exploratory study. *International Journal of Nursing Studies, 23*, 315–323.

Schorr, J. (1993). Music and pattern change in chronic pain. *Advances in Nursing Science, 15*, 27–36.

Tabloski, P.A., McKinnon-Howe, L., & Remington, R. (1995, January/February). Effects of calming music on the level of agitation in cognitively impaired nursing home residents. *American Journal of Alzheimer's Care and Related Disorders & Research*, pp. 10–15.

10

Activities as an Intervention for Disturbed Behaviors on the Dementia-Specific Care Unit

Linda L. Buettner, Ph.D., C.T.R.S.

The management of disturbed behaviors in older adults with dementia is a common problem that represents one of the major challenges for activities professionals on the dementia-specific care unit (DSCU). Such management requires them to take on an important role and a new way of thinking about activities programming. The activities specialist for the DSCU must master the cognitive and behavioral signs and symptoms of dementia and create an assortment of diversional and therapeutic programs to meet the unique needs of residents with dementia.

The primary goal of this chapter is to assist the activities professional in providing activities for residents of the DSCU that lead to increased positive behaviors and decreased negative behaviors. Information is presented to help the activities specialist to 1) understand some of the symptoms and what their impact is on the provision of activities, 2) identify the specific behaviors manifested and understand why the behavior may have occurred, and 3) design a program of therapeutic and diversional activities to meet the specific needs of the residents.

SYMPTOMS OF DEMENTIA

A set of symptoms, known as the four A's—amnesia, aphasia, agnosia, and apraxia (Powers, 1996)—affects every part of the lives of people with dementia, even their leisure-time activities. Amnesia, or memory loss, is the first symptom that occurs in the disease process. People with dementia initially experience short-term memory loss. Gradually, long-term memory is also affected. People with dementia may forget what they just said, the names and faces of other people involved, how to get to an activity, or what to do when they get there. Aphasia is often the second symptom in the disease process. Aphasia alters the ability to use and understand words. This communication deficit makes socializing difficult, understanding directions problematic, and making needs known during an activity extremely frustrating for the people affected. Agnosia is the third symptom of which the activities professional should be aware. This symptom affects residents' ability to recognize and use familiar objects. People with dementia may not know what to do with recreation equipment or other common materials unless retaught or demonstrated each time they want to use them. The final symptom with which the activities professional should be familiar is apraxia. Apraxia alters the ability to perform once-familiar motor skills and gradually leads to extreme physical disability. Because of these motor problems people with dementia gradually need greater amounts of physical assistance during activities programs, and their risk for falls, contractures, and loss of independent leisure-time functioning increases.

Although the signs and symptoms of dementia may be similar from one older adult to another, there are a variety of causes for negative behaviors, including dementia itself. For that reason, the activities specialist on the DSCU should become conversant with each resident's diagnosis and its implications. Although Alzheimer's disease, vascular dementia, and Lewy bodies disease all are associated with behavioral disturbances, individuals with these dementing disorders do not necessarily decline at the same rate or follow the same trajectory of disease progression (Geldmacher, 1996). The behavior displayed by individuals with these diseases also varies as the result of a host of other factors such as functional abilities, perceived environmental stressors, and personal needs. In other words, "if you've met one person with [dementia], you've only met one person with [dementia]" (Bell & Troxel, 1997, p. 5). An understanding of each resident's diagnosis and his or her behavior patterns is an intricate first step in determining the appropriate approach to behavior management.

PASSIVITY: A MULTIDISCIPLINARY PROBLEM

Frequently, the nursing facility resident with dementia assumes the role of a dependent or passive participant in his or her care, treatment, and life itself. The resident receives his or her prescribed care plan and all too often is not encour-

aged to participate actively. Personal care providers may feel that it is more efficient to dress, bathe, or perform an activity of daily living for the individual than
to allow the time, structure, and the cueing necessary for the resident to complete
the task independently (Vogelpohl, Beck, Heacock, & Mercer, 1996). The same
phenomenon occurs in recreational activities. Many times, activities programs are
evaluated in terms of numbers of attendees rather than in terms of the level of
involvement or therapeutic outcomes achieved (Buettner & Martin, 1994). This
misguided evaluation leads to large-group programs, too much or too little stimulation, and not enough individual attention for each resident with dementia
(Buettner, 1994). Thus, the activity program becomes part of the problem instead
of a therapeutic intervention. In both examples, the facility staff takes on a much
more active role than does the individual with dementia. The result is that residents with dementia prematurely lose control, motivation, and skills.

Human beings are active, living organisms who derive satisfaction from
using their innate abilities, and people with dementia are no exception (Butcher,
Shiver, & Butcher, 1984). Research shows that active involvement in structured
activities significantly reduces boredom, agitation, and other behavior problems
(Aronstein, Olsen, & Schulman, 1996; Buettner, 1994; Buettner, Lundegren,
Lago, Farrell, & Smith, 1996; Rabinovich & Cohen-Mansfield, 1991). Other
studies have demonstrated that therapeutic recreation can lead to a reduction in
falls (Buettner, Kernan, & Carroll, 1990; Buettner & Waitkvicz, in press), less
noise- and stress-related agitation in residents on the DSCU, and less depression
in the residents involved (Buettner & Ferrario, 1998). Rovner, Steele, Shmuely,
and Folstein (1996) found that residents who were involved in a structured program of activities designed specifically for individuals with dementia were more
likely to participate in activities, less likely to be restrained, and far less likely to
need psychotropic medications.

BEHAVIOR DISTURBANCES OF
OLDER ADULTS WITH DEMENTIA

Researchers and clinicians have attempted to define, qualify, and quantify the
negative behaviors of individuals with dementia. Many different terms have been
used and a variety of assessment tools developed to approach these tasks. For the
purposes of this chapter the behaviors are examined across a broad spectrum that
includes positive as well as negative behaviors (see Figure 1). Behavior along the
spectrum may or may not be linear (i.e., residents may go from one behavior to
another in a matter of minutes without passing through the other behaviors along
the line). However, a resident may get stuck at a given point along the spectrum,
and his or her behavior disturbance may become habitual. This spectrum of
behaviors is simply a visual tool used to help the activities specialist identify or
name behaviors.

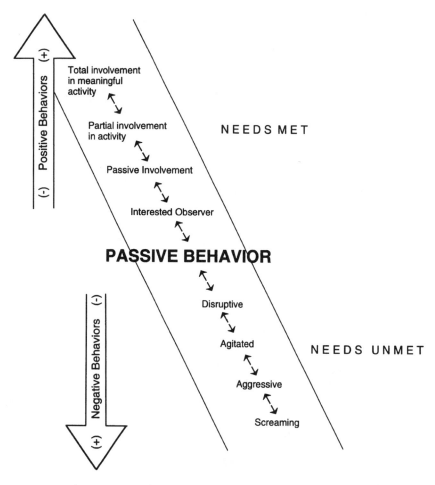

Figure 1.   The spectrum of behaviors in older adults with dementia who are residents of DSCUs.

Often, positive behaviors are observed when a resident takes part in activity that is meaningful and appropriate to his or her level of functioning. Residents in the positive portion of the spectrum engage in activities that match their abilities and interests. They have the opportunity to practice, use, and maintain skills. Residents experience enjoyment, a sense of accomplishment, an opportunity for self-expression, or companionship, which leads to an enhanced quality of life. Differing degrees of involvement occur on the positive side of the spectrum. For example, one resident may be watching and enjoying a game of tetherball as a spectator. He may give advice sporadically or cheer for others. Another resident may be sitting at the same table with others taking part in a modified game of dominoes. This resident may enjoy keeping score or pointing out openings to others. Another resident may wander throughout the activity trail on the DSCU, occasionally stopping to pick up a recreational item, look at it, and carry it off to another location. On the far side of the DSCU six residents may bake an apple pie in a cooking program with assistance from the activities therapist. Engagement in age- and stage-appropriate activities, to whatever degree, leads to positive behavior on this spectrum.

Negative behaviors also are manifested in various degrees or intensities. Passive behavior is a negative symptom of dementia in which residents remain inactive and uninvolved for long periods of time. Although many health care providers do not view passivity as a problem behavior, it can lead to isolation, sensory deprivation, and potential disuse syndrome (Carpenito, 1991; Galynker, Roane, Miner, Feinberg, & Watts, 1995). Moreover, residents who are inactive for extended periods often lose skills because of atrophy in addition to those lost as a result of the disease process (Buettner, 1988).

Agitation is the broad term used commonly in describing behavior disturbances and is defined as inappropriate verbal, vocal, or motor activity (Cohen-Mansfield & Belig, 1986). Agitated behavior has been described as arising from numerous causes and manifesting as disruptive, abusive, or aggressive behavior toward self, others, or objects in the environment (Middleton, Richardson, & Berman, 1997). Displaying appropriate behavior with inappropriate frequency also has been described as a negative behavior in the literature. Many residents of DSCUs display varying degrees of disruptive repetitive sounds, words, or movements. Screaming is categorized separately on this spectrum because it seems to have a different cause and a serious impact on all who live, work, or take part in activities on the DSCU. Any of the disruptive behaviors described here may intensify into a more serious level of agitation or aggression, as in the following vignette:

> A resident of the DSCU sits near the nurse's station, repeating, "I want to go home. I want to go home." Another resident picks at her own clothing and rocks back and forth quietly. Several other residents appear to be sleeping, slumped over in their chairs. A recently toileted resident begins to moan and scream intermittently. The sleeping residents awaken. Several individuals become agitated and yell "Shut up! Shut up!" at her. One resident reaches across another to hit the disruptive woman.

The vignette shows that behaviors can change within seconds or minutes and that they can have many different causes or triggers. Some of the disruptive behaviors mentioned in the vignette appear to be the result of boredom and lack of stimulation. Noise triggered agitated behaviors in several members of the passively sleeping group, which led to an aggressive incident.

Facility staff should evaluate a resident's needs for activity, stimulation, and rest as soon as he or she is admitted to the DSCU. Positive and negative behavior patterns can easily be plotted to indicate the times when needs are either met or unmet. Figure 2 follows the behavior pattern of a new resident during the first 24

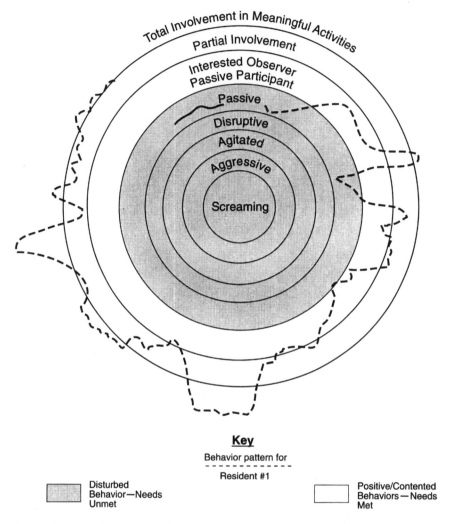

Figure 2. Circular pattern of behavior, showing peaks and valleys of disturbed and positive behaviors.

hours after admission to a DSCU. In the following scenario, staff intervene using activities, and the outcome is very different from that of the earlier vignette.

Mrs. M's family left her sitting quietly and passively watching others near the nurse's station after her admission to the facility was completed. The activities therapist and the nurse manager worked together to engage Mrs. M. in the weekly 30s–40s dance program that was under way in the lounge. Initially, Mrs. M. just watched and smiled, but gradually, she became more involved, first requesting a song, then getting up to dance after a few minutes. At lunchtime, Mrs. M. volunteered to set the table, but became upset, sad, and withdrawn after the meal. A staff member noticed her isolation and asked her to join the Editorial Group, which was planning the next issue of the DSCU's newspaper. She joined the group, listening passively. When the group reached the "New Resident" section of the paper, a participant suggested interviewing Mrs. M. During the interview Mrs. M. took the opportunity to talk about her life losses and the move to the nursing facility. Most important, she connected with another resident during the group program, and the two new friends walked off, talking, after the program ended.

The positive and negative behaviors of older adults with dementia evolve daily across the behavior spectrum. If staff does not take the time necessary to engage residents in activities their behaviors may deteriorate into those falling in the negative realm of the spectrum.

CAUSES OF BEHAVIOR DISTURBANCES

Rather than viewing a behavior disturbance as a psychiatric symptom of dementia, it may be appropriate for the activities professional and staff to think of the behavior as an unmet need that the individual is trying to express or his or her pursuit of a goal (Algase et al., 1996). Factors within the person, the immediate environment, or both, influence the individual's behavior. These factors are dynamic, and thus behaviors may vary based on the situation or the individual's history. For example, wandering may be related to a lifetime of relieving stress by physical means (Coltharp, Richie, & Kass, 1996); repetitive vocalizing with words may be a plea for opportunities to socialize (White, Kass, & Richie, 1996); screaming or moaning may indicate depression or pain (White et al., 1996); and repetitive rubbing, picking, or noisemaking may indicate a need for sensory stimulation (Buettner et al., 1990). Most behavior has an underlying meaning, and the activities professional must try to determine that meaning before providing an intervention to the behavior. Simply prescribing and administering psychotropic medications for the resident experiencing behavior disturbances does little to address the true need of the whole person and ignores the message the individual is attempting to convey.

A primary cause of negative behaviors is boredom. Research to examine the link between unoccupied time of residents of nursing facilities as a cause for agitation was conducted at a large metropolitan nursing facility (Cohen-Mansfield, Werner, & Marx, 1992). Members of the facility's nursing staff felt that boredom triggered the behavior disturbances in 54.9% of the 144 residents studied. After this preliminary study of staff, the research team studied the relationship between agitation and boredom in a small group of residents. Observational data on time use and behavior disorders revealed the ways that residents typically spent their time. Using a stratified random time-sampling method, 24 residents were observed for 3 minutes per hour during waking hours for 3 months. The researchers found that residents were unoccupied 63% of the time they were observed. Further data analysis revealed that residents manifested greater numbers of agitated behaviors when they were unoccupied and fewer agitated behaviors when involved in structured activities.

The influence of other factors such as functional abilities, environmental stressors, and the personal needs of people with dementia on their behavior also must be understood. These factors can be stable for long periods of time or can change frequently. Therefore, the activities specialist should make a quick assessment of residents' needs and their affect each time the residents are involved in a program (Lawton, Van Haitsma, & Klapper, 1996). With this information, the activities specialist can adjust the approach he or she uses, his or her communication style, or the expectations of the residents. The activities specialist should establish flexible activities areas and program structures that provide the appropriate amount of stimulation and challenge; the appropriate amount is based on the quick assessment completed earlier in the program. Therapeutic programming environments play an important role in outcomes (Buettner et al., 1996). Residents of DSCUs experience the most success in small-group programs, with reduced noise from outside sources and with opportunities for movement and socialization.

THERAPEUTIC AND DIVERSIONAL ACTIVITIES PROGRAMMING

Two general types of programs are necessary in order to manage the behavior disorders of residents of DSCUs. First, a structured program of therapeutic activities should be designed with the intent of attaining specific goals and objectives in each resident's care plan. These activities are based on assessment of the individual and are facilitated by a therapist or activities specialist. The second type of program needed on the DSCU is an assortment of diversional activities. Diversional activities are used to refocus residents' attention, calm or comfort residents, promote independence, or prevent boredom. Diversional activities should be available throughout the DSCU and all staff should be encouraged to use them as interventions. Both types of activities, therapeutic and diversional, are needed to maintain a high quality of life for residents who cannot structure their own leisure time (Buettner & Martin, 1995).

Assessment is the first step in high-quality activities programming and should include cognitive and physical functioning as well as the past leisure interests of each resident (Buettner & Martin, 1995). It is particularly important to note whether the residents are immobile or unable to seek out stimulation, have hearing or visual impairments, or seem to be experiencing psychological distress because of pain or depression. Specific activities guidelines for these problem areas are highlighted in Table 1. The activities specialist also should select tools to measure residents' progress in cognitive areas, mood, behaviors, and general functional

Table 1.   Specific needs to address, expression of needs, and suggested interventions

Need	Behaviors that may be observed	Suggested interventions
Understimulated	Repetitive picking, tapping, or rubbing Takes apart clothing, stuffed animals Repetitive noises (e.g., "na-na-na") Creates own stimulation Grabs on or pulls others nearby	Small-group social activity Sensory integration Food preparation groups Locate near activity centers Use headphones, animal-assisted (pet) therapy Simple Pleasures, tactile items
Overstimulated	Anxious or tense Yells "Help me!" or "Get me out of here!" Tries to get away Appears desperate Hits, pushes, kicks at others	Use calming music or relaxation One staff member only communicates Relocate in quieter area, do not isolate Phone calls from family or friends Nature activities or flower arranging
Immobile	Frustration and repetitive words or movements Struggles or feels uncomfortable Spatial disorientation Excessive passivity	Hands and feet stimulation, sensory hand washing Reposition for programs, place feet on floor Locate near activity centers and place recreational items within reach Sensory integration, opportunities for movement and exercise Therapeutic food preparation group
Restless	Paces Wanders Pulls down decorations Shakes doors and tries to get out	Ambulation program Activity fitness trail/Leisure lounge Wanderer's cart to push Simple Pleasures—wave machine or squeezies Finger foods and drinks to carry

(continued)

Table 1—*continued*

Need	Behaviors that may be observed	Suggested interventions
Depressed	Weeps, cries, screams Refuses food, drinks, medications, group activities Isolates self—passive and withdrawn	One-to-one activities Spiritual activities—music Use reminiscence and the familiar Reassure frequently—feelings group Hot water bottle in a blanket Exercise and walking Animal-assisted therapy Psychiatric evaluation/treatment for depression
Fatigued	Irritable and short tempered Complains Slumps in chair or slides out Passive for extended periods	Reduce stimulation in program area Control length of activities/visits Provide relaxation programs (e.g., air mat therapy) Reposition in beanbag chair Schedule rest periods
Stress relief (psychological)	Worries, refuses to leave room Cries, asks for help repeatedly Paranoia Screams	Safe, calm environment and familiar routine Comfort with touch—use hot water bottle Watch videotape of loved ones Verbal reassurance—talk one-to-one Medical evaluation for pain

fitness during programs. This information should be gathered regularly to demonstrate the efficacy of the interventions. It is also important to obtain information from residents and their families, and friends or companions about activity likes and dislikes, personality traits, and past coping mechanisms (Buettner & Martin, 1995). A leisure interest profile should then be used to examine past involvement with hobbies, games, social interests, outdoor pursuits, and cultural events.

After assessment data are gathered, therapeutic and diversional activities programs are designed to match the residents' level of functioning, needs, and interests. The therapeutic recreation programs can be categorized into three major areas: adapted recreation, leisure education, and therapy (Peterson & Gunn, 1984). Examples of the three types of programs follow:

Adapted recreation
   Open recreation in leisure lounge or activities areas
   Adapted bowling or bocce league
   Special recreational events
   Gardening/adapted gardening
   Free-time kitchen activities (e.g., doing dishes, setting/clearing the table, preparing snacks)
   Computer games/table games (i.e., games that are played while sitting at a table)
   Community recreational outings (e.g., shopping, lunch, community events)
   Pets/photography club/dance club/other hobbies

Leisure education
   Leisure education for staff and families
   Signage directing residents to activities
   Re-education of residents on how to use recreational items
   "Leisurely Look Newsletter" program to raise awareness of recreational opportunities and self-expression

Recreational therapy
   Air mat therapy
   Exercise-to-music therapy
   Sensory integration
   Stimulation of hands and feet
   Cognitive stimulation and feelings group
   Afternoon social skills programs with families
   Falls prevention program
   Morning walking group
   Balance and strength group
   Therapeutic cooking groups
   Pancake cooking club
   Blender snacks group (puréed diets)
   Finger foods socials
   Weekend apple pie bakers
   Gross motor arts and crafts group

An important consideration in creating an activities program is scheduling the particular activities designed for the DSCU. Each DSCU experiences certain times during the day, evening, or night in which greater numbers of negative behaviors occur. Activities should be planned to fit the unit's routine and provide structure and intervention options when these clusters of negative behaviors take place. The therapeutic activities programs should fit into the unit timetable of care activities already in place (Buettner & Ferrario, 1998). Studies demonstrate that to enhance participation, therapeutic activities programming should mesh with other unit activities, not compete with them (Buettner & Ferrario, 1998; Voelkl, Galecki, & Fries, 1996). For example, programs of interest to particular residents should be set up around their bath or physical therapy schedule in order to avoid conflicts.

Beyond individual schedules, each DSCU experiences periods of high need, when recreation therapy sessions can be helpful. For example, often, the early morning hours between rising and breakfast are a time when falls occur (Commodore, 1995). These hours are an ideal time to schedule a structured walking or falls prevention program. Another high-need time is at change of shift. A program that draws residents' attention away from the nurses' station at shift changes can be helpful. Also beneficial is the delivery of mail and messages to residents at an activity center set up at the far end of the DSCU. Figure 3 shows a sample of an integrated unit schedule. Transitions between programs are also high-need times and must be scheduled carefully, with nursing services in mind (Buettner & Ferrario, 1998). When a structured program ends, residents should not be left sitting with nothing to do. All staff should be trained to provide a recreational item of the resident's choice to the resident when completing care. For example, as the exercise-to-music therapy program ends, residents can be given a magazine to read or sewing card to use independently while waiting for the distribution of refreshments. Also, often, residents are brought to the dining room and seated at tables with nothing to do until the meal is served: Sensory tablecloths should be used with lower-functioning residents, higher-functioning residents should be asked to help set tables, and other residents should be provided with individual basins and sponges for a sensory hand-washing program. Index card files of "things to do" can be created and placed strategically in the dining room, nurses' station, and activities center (see Figure 4 for suggestions) for times when staff cannot think of an activity.

CONSIDERATIONS FOR THERAPEUTIC ACTIVITIES PROGRAMMING

Researchers have demonstrated efficacy for a specific type of therapeutic activities programming called neurodevelopmental sequencing (NDSP). NDSP not only reduces negative behaviors but also improves specific areas of functioning related to strength, flexibility, and mobility (Buettner et al., 1990; Buettner & Ferrario, 1998; Buettner, Lundegren, Lago, Farrell, & Smith, 1996). The program uses assessment data and principles taken from neurodevelopmental theory and sensory integration to address residents' leisure time challenges through a variety of sensorimotor activities (Buettner, 1988, 1994). The goals of NDSP are to improve

6:00–8:00	CNA—Bathing 1, or Dressing and Grooming Program—Resident rooms RT—Morning Walking Groups and Falls Prevention—Hallways to Dining Room Nursing—Morning Hydration and Health Assessment—Dining Room
8:00–9:00	Breakfast Groups—Dining Room RT—Pancake Cooking Group Nursing and CNA—Cultured Diners Group Nursing and CNA—Finger Foods Group/Assisted Diners Group
9:00–9:30	CNA—Continence Program 1 CNA, SW, Housekeeping—Assist residents to activities centers— Set up activities
9:30–10:00	RT—Exercise-to-music therapy Public radio show—Activity center 1 Volunteer pet care—Activity center 2 CNA—Nails and hair—Activity center 3
10:00–10:30	CNA—Continence Program 2 CNA—Bathing 2 Nourishment (juices and finger food snacks) pass
10:30–11:30	RT—Air mat therapy program for exercise Nursing—Dancing and music in activity room Volunteers—Simple Pleasure items at activity centers 1–3
11:30–12:00	Pre-lunch activities in dining room CNA—Sensory Tablecloths Group AD—Table Setting Group COTA from rehab. dept.—Sensory Hand Washing Group
12:00–1:00	Lunch program—CNA and Nursing Outdoor Cafe Dining Group (nice weather) Finger Food Picnic Group
1:00–1:30	CNA–Continence Program 3 Housekeeping, SW, ADON—Assist residents to activity centers— Set up activities
1:30–2:30	Volunteer Activity Aides—Adapted Bowling League RT and Nursing—Leisurely Look Newsletter group Afternoon rest period
2:30–3:00	Nourishments and juices RT and COTA—Snack Group—Prepare your own afternoon snack CNA and Families—Outdoor walks or Walk-the-Dog Program
3:00–4:00	Volunteer and RT—Mail and Messages Group Visiting Musician Program
4:00–4:30	CNA—Continence Program 4 Leisure Lounge—Recreation of choice with afterschool volunteers/families Feelings Group—Activity center 2 Resident piano playing—Activity center 3
4:30–5:15	Pre-dinner programming in dining room RT—The Price is Right Cognitive Game CNA—Sensory Tablecloths Group COTA—Sensory Hand-Washing Group
5:30–6:30	Dinner Groups
6:30–9:00	Family and friends activities programs CNA—Rolling bedtime preparation CNA—Bathtime 3

Figure 3.   Sample integrated program schedule.

Give out mail and messages—help residents write response
Activity walker—help a resident take a walk using the activity walker
Take resident for a walk outdoors or around the sensory trail
Fold towels or ball socks
Fix-it bin—give resident bin of stuff to tinker with
Activity tablecloth—spread out on a table for 3–4 residents to use
Drawing or painting with materials from expressive arts bin
Flower arranging
Videotape of family/friends and discussion
Large cards or dominoes
Dancing to 30s, 40s tunes
Tether volleyball game with 2–5 residents
Table ball game
Reading program
Bowling for dollars—use "fun" money to play
Sewing cards
Hairbrushing
Dusting or cleaning
Apply hand lotion
Tic-tac-toe game
Give out "Simple Pleasures" items
    Activity purse or tackle box
    Polarfleece butterfly or fish
    Wave machine
    Message magnet game
    Test your strength game
    Squeezies
    Home decorator books
    Activity vest or muff
Exercise bands/music
The Price is Right game

Figure 4.   Activity ideas for index card files.

residents' strength, flexibility, ability to move about, and ability to make leisure choices. Residents who have taken part in this program have demonstrated dramatic improvements in both physical and psychological areas: Negative behaviors diminished significantly in all participants (Buettner et al., 1996).

In addition to the type of activities provided, group size and task difficulty are important considerations for the activities specialist. Residents with dementia need small-group activities that are based on their level of functioning (Buettner et al., 1996). Residents attending the group should understand the meaning of what they are doing and be able to participate actively (Voelkl, 1990). If the activity is too difficult residents will become frustrated; if the activity is too easy residents may become bored and may fail to benefit or wander away. If there is excessive noise or confusion, agitation may result (Hall & Buckwalter, 1987). The activities facilitator must understand that it is the active involvement of residents that is important, not the finished product (Buettner & Martin, 1995).

Therapeutic activities programming should be designed to help residents maintain or improve their level of functioning (Buettner & Martin, 1995). In this vein, a wellness or preventive component such as fall prevention can be added to therapeutic activities programs (Buettner & Waitkavicz, in press). These programs should provide activities that help residents maintain their ability to walk, talk, and eat independently. Programs that enhance balance, strength, flexibility, use of upper extremities, and self-expression are essential to maintaining older adults' daily living skills (Kemp & Mitchell, 1992). The focus of therapeutic activities programs should be sensorimotor, with many opportunities for free movement, simple choices, and expression of feelings (Buettner, 1994).

Residents should be reassessed every 10–12 weeks. The tasks in the therapeutic activities program must be refined constantly to meet the ever-changing needs of residents.

CONSIDERATIONS FOR DIVERSIONAL ACTIVITIES PROGRAMMING

Preliminary research has demonstrated that diversional recreational interventions are useful in defusing agitation and reducing boredom in nursing facility residents with dementia (Aronstein, Olsen, & Schulman, 1996). Residents who are not scheduled for a small-group therapeutic recreation program also need activities. To meet their needs, safe age- and stage-appropriate recreational items should be set up and made available at various locations throughout the DSCU. If space is available, a leisure lounge stocked with interesting independent activities (see Figure 5 for suggestions) can be set up by DSCU staff and families. A mobile leisure cart is also recommended for residents who prefer to stay in their rooms (Buettner & Martin, 1995; Voelkl et al., 1996). Some residents enjoy pushing the cart around the unit and providing recreational items to others (Buettner & Greenstein, 1997).

A diversional activities program called Simple Pleasures is being studied in DSCUs in three upstate New York nursing facilities (Buettner & Greenstein, 1997). This program involved designing 30 inexpensive, easy-to-make recreational items for individuals with dementia. After pilot testing the items for safety and resident preferences, plans and patterns were developed for each of the items so that families, nursing facilities, and community volunteers could fabricate the items for the residents. A large notebook holds a set of simple directions for each item, which is available for staff and visitors' use. The goal is to make available a myriad of easy-to-make and easy-to-use sensorimotor interventions to residents, staff, and families.

In addition to the availability of diversional recreational items, staff training is critical. All staff members should understand that it is important to assist resi-

Simple Pleasures items	Exercise resources
Art materials	Walking mile chart
Activity purses/briefcase	Therabands
Tackle boxes	Weight jugs
Wave machine	Ribbons
Message magnet sets	Balloons
Home decorator books	Air mat
Fabric balls	Sports
Activity tablecloth	Nerf basketball
Activity vest	Putting green
Activity aprons	Shuffleboard
Wall-mounted activities: fishing, playing	Bocce
ring game, flower arranging, and	Horseshoes
hanging laundry	Tetherball
Music resources	Nerf football
Headphones with Walkman/keyboard	Table games
Collection of music and stories on tape	Large face cards
Songbooks	Large dominoes
Bells/drums	Board games (no small pieces)
Stereo system	Tablecloth checkers/tic-tac-toe
Piano or keyboard	Pinball
Black paper/chalk	Other
Nontoxic paints	Magazines/books
Large brushes	Catalogs
Nontoxic clay	Junk mail
Paper of various colors/textures	Dresser of stuff to rummage through
Old greeting cards	Remote control jeep
Yarn, ribbon, etc.	

Figure 5.   Leisure lounge or mobile cart materials.

dents to the activities centers located throughout the DSCU and to set up the activity that is scheduled. For example, after meals residents can be guided to small activity centers set up at the end of hallways to listen to a story on tape, a radio broadcast, or a classical music concert. Others can take part in a tetherball game in the leisure lounge. Another small group might receive a visit from a volunteer musician or have an opportunity to interact with pets. Higher-functioning residents often enjoy taking charge of these programs at the various activities centers. A large daily activities schedule of residents' names and the various programs should be posted in the dining room and near the nurses' station so that all staff know where residents should go. This schedule also helps staff handle the concern from residents, "I don't know what to do."

. . .

In both therapeutic and diversional activities programming, consistency balanced with flexibility must be maintained. If residents need calming, staff must adjust the program with that goal in mind. Programs should not be canceled for the convenience of staff. Above all, open communication between the nurse manager and the activities specialist is essential. A constant relay of information about resident health issues, appointments, and other concerns leads to the most suitable program opportunities.

CONCLUSION

The activities specialist on the DSCU has the exciting, important, and challenging task of designing programs that make a difference in residents' and caregivers' lives. It is clear from the research that residents need abundant opportunities for movement, stimulation, self-expression, socialization, and relaxation. Structuring such programs requires the activities specialist to develop and use expert clinical skills and creative strategies. Accurate behavior assessment is essential to the development of the activities care plan and to the daily provision of activities programs. The activities specialist must realize that because of the cognitive changes caused by dementia, changing environmental stimuli, and fluctuations in behavior from medications, residents of DSCUs may react differently from one program to the next. Activity specialists who provide services on a DSCU must be sensitive, flexible, innovative, and attentive to residents' needs.

An innovative and integrated activities program that provides both therapeutic and diversional options to all residents can add meaning and good quality to life on a DSCU. Structuring the special care environment so that residents feel free to make leisure time choices, have autonomy, perceive rewards, gain confidence, and use remaining physical skills safely is essential to enhancing their quality of life. Having a repertoire of effective activities to use as behavioral interventions reduces residents' negative behaviors and provides staff with opportunities to use alternative strategies. The most important outcomes are that each resident is active and involved in life and his or her behavior problem is managed with a minimum of psychotropic medications.

REFERENCES

Algase, D., Beck, C., Kolanowski, A., Whall, A., Berent, S., Richards, K., & Beattie, E. (1996). "Need-driven dementia-compromised behavior": An alternative view of disruptive behavior. *American Journal of Alzheimer's Disease, 11*(6), 10–19.

Aronstein, Z., Olsen, R., & Schulman, E. (1996). The nursing assistant's use of recreational interventions for behavioral management of residents with Alzheimer's disease. *American Journal of Alzheimer's Disease, 11,* 32–39.

Bell, V., & Troxel, D. (1997). *The best friends approach to Alzheimer's care.* Baltimore: Health Professions Press.

Buettner, L. (1988). Utilizing developmental theory and adapted equipment with regressed geriatric patients in therapeutic recreation. *Therapeutic Recreation Journal, 22*(3), 72–79.

Buettner, L. (1994). *Therapeutic recreation as an intervention for persons with dementia and agitation: An efficacy study*. Unpublished doctoral dissertation. The Pennsylvania State University, University Park.

Buettner, L., & Ferrario, J. (1998). *A therapeutic intervention for nursing home residents with dementia*. National Alzheimer's Association Pilot Research Grant No. PRG 94-022. Chicago: Alzheimer's Association.

Buettner, L., & Greenstein, D. (1997). Simple Pleasures: A multi-level sensorimotor intervention for nursing home residents with dementia. Albany: New York State Department of Health Dementia Research Grant.

Buettner, L., Kernan, B., & Carroll, G. (1990). Therapeutic recreation for the frail elderly: A new approach. In G.L. Hitzhusen & J.R. Gigstad (Eds.), *Global therapeutic recreation I. Selected papers from the 1st International Symposium on Therapeutic Recreation* (pp. 82–88). Columbia: University of Missouri Press.

Buettner, L., Lundegren, H., Lago, D., Farrell, P., & Smith, R. (1996). Therapeutic recreation as an intervention for persons with dementia and agitation. *American Journal of Alzheimer's Disease, 11,* 4–12.

Buettner, L., & Martin, S. (1994). Never too old, too sick, or too bad for therapeutic recreation: A biopsychosocial approach. In G.L. Hitzhusen & J.R. Gigstad (Eds.), *Global therapeutic recreation III. Selected papers from the 3rd International Symposium on Therapeutic Recreation* (pp. 135–139). Columbia: University of Missouri Press.

Buettner, L., & Martin, S. (1995). *Therapeutic recreation for the nursing home*. State College, PA: Venture Publishing.

Buettner, L., & Waitkavicz, J. (in press). Falls as a constraint to leisure among older adults. In G.L. Hitzhusen (Ed.), *Global therapeutic recreation V. Selected papers from the 5th International Symposium on Therapeutic Recreation*. Columbia: University of Missouri Press.

Butcher, C., Shiver, J., & Butcher, R. (1984). *Recreation for society*. Englewood Cliffs, NJ: Prentice Hall.

Carpenito, L. (1991). *Handbook of nursing diagnosis* (4th ed.). Philadelphia: J.B. Lippincott.

Cohen-Mansfield, J., & Belig, N. (1996). Agitated behaviors in the elderly: A conceptual review. *Journal of the American Geriatrics Society, 34,* 711–721.

Cohen-Mansfield, J., Werner, P., & Marx, M. (1992). Observational data on time use and behavior problems in the nursing home. *Journal of Applied Gerontology, 11,* 114–117.

Coltharp, W., Richie, M., & Kass, M. (1996). Wandering. *Journal of Gerontological Nursing, 22*(11), 5–10.

Commodore, D. (1995). Falls in the elderly population: A look at incidence, risks, health care costs, and preventative strategies. *Rehabilitation Nursing, 20,* 84–89.

Galynker, I., Roane, D., Miner, C., Feinberg, T., & Watts, P. (1995). Negative symptoms in patients with Alzheimer's disease. *American Journal of Geriatric Psychiatry, 3*(1), 52–59.

Geldmacher, D. (1996). Dementia: An overview of types. *Current Approaches to Dementia, 2*(1), 1–2.

Hall, G., & Buckwalter, K. (1987). Progressively lowered stress threshold: A conceptual model for care of adults with Alzheimer's disease. *Archives of Psychiatric Nursing, 1,* 399–406.

Kemp, B., & Mitchell, J. (1992). Functional assessment in geriatric mental health. In J. Birren, B. Sloan, & G. Cohen (Eds.), *Handbook of mental health and aging* (pp. 671–697). San Diego, CA: San Diego Press.

Lawton, P., Van Haitsma, K., & Klapper, J. (1996). Observed affect in nursing home residents with Alzheimer's disease. *Journal of Gerontology, 51B*(1), 3–12.

Middleton, J., Richardson, J., & Berman, E. (1997). An assessment and intervention study of aggressive behavior in cognitively impaired institutionalized elderly. *American Journal of Alzheimer's Disease, 12*(1), 24–29.

Peterson, C.A., & Gunn, S.L. (1984). *Therapeutic recreation program design: Principles and procedures.* Englewood Cliffs, NJ: Prentice Hall.

Powers, R. (1996, May). *Nurse aides: The real foot soldiers in the nursing home.* Paper presented at The Art of Alzheimer's Care in the Nursing Home Conference, Birmingham, AL.

Rabinovich, B., & Cohen-Mansfield, J. (1991). *The impact of participation in structured recreational activities on the agitated behavior of nursing home residents: An observational study.* Research Monograph 60. Rockville, MD: Hebrew Home of Greater Washington.

Rovner, B., Steele, C., Shmuely, Y., & Folstein, J. (1996). A randomized trial of dementia care in nursing homes. *Journal of the American Geriatrics Society, 44*, 7–13.

Voelkl, J.E. (1990). The challenge skill ratio of daily experiences among older adults residing in nursing homes. *Therapeutic Recreation Journal, 24*, 7–17.

Voelkl, J., Galecki, A., & Fries, B. (1996). Nursing home residents with severe cognitive impairments: Predictors of participation in activity groups. *Therapeutic Recreation Journal, 30*, 27–40.

Vogelpohl, T., Beck, C., Heacock, P., & Mercer, S. (1996). I can do it! Dressing: Promoting independence through individualized strategies. *Journal of Gerontological Nursing, 22*(3), 39–46.

White, M., Kass, M., & Richie, M. (1996). Vocally disruptive behavior. *Journal of Gerontological Nursing, 22*(11), 23–39.

11

Nonpharmacological Approaches to the Management of the Behavioral Consequences of Advanced Dementia

Ladislav Volicer, M.D., Ph.D., Ellen Mahoney, D.NSc., R.N. C.S., and
Elizabeth J. Brown, R.D.H., M.S.

The prevalence of progressive dementias increases with age and reaches beyond 70% in older adults living in nursing facilities (Chandler & Chandler, 1988; Rovner, Kafonek, & Filipp, 1986). No effective treatment stops or reverses the progression of these diseases, although some drugs temporarily improve a person's functions or decrease the rate of progression of dementia (Knapp et al., 1994; Paganini-Hill & Henderson, 1996; Rogers et al., 1996; Sano et al., 1997). Several forms of progressive dementias are known, but the same management approaches can be used because the dementias often occur in combination and have similar behavioral consequences.

BEHAVIORAL CONSEQUENCES OF DEMENTIA

The behavioral consequences of progressive dementias are either disruptive or nondisruptive. Although most studies concentrate on disruptive behaviors because they affect other residents and staff, a nondisruptive behavior disorder is also important from the point of view of the individual with dementia. Nondisruptive behavior disorders are exhibited most commonly as apathy or withdrawal. People with dementia often isolate themselves in their rooms and refuse to participate in activities. They may also refuse food, medications, or both.

Disruptive behaviors are very common, occurring in up to 87% of residents of nursing facilities (Cohen-Mansfield, 1988; Ryden, Bossenmaier, & McLachlan, 1991). Most authors combine these behaviors under the single label "agitation, combativeness, or aggression." However, it is useful to differentiate between two types of disruptive behavior, provoked or unprovoked, because each requires different interventions for its optimal management. Most disruptive behavior is provoked, either by environmental stimuli (e.g., noise, temperature extremes) or by contact with another individual. Provoked disruptive behavior is observed most commonly during direct caregiving that involves touching (Ryden & Feldt, 1992). The most common cause is confusion about and lack of understanding by the person with dementia as to why he or she needs to be touched or to receive care. The person with dementia tries to resist caregiving efforts, and if the caregiver persists the person tries to defend him- or herself and may even strike out. Resistance to care is the underlying cause of provoked disruptive behavior because, if left alone, older adults with progressive dementias are rarely aggressive. Therefore, it is useful to call this disruptive behavior "resistiveness."

The term "agitation" is best reserved for an unprovoked disruptive behavior. Agitation may be defined as "those patient behaviors that communicate to others that the patient is experiencing an unpleasant state of excitement" (Hurley et al., 1995, p. 161). Agitation may be either physical (e.g., restlessness, fidgeting) or verbal (e.g., repeated vocalizations). For the behavior to be considered unprovoked, it cannot be related to physical needs of the person with dementia that can be remedied. Thus, it is important to exclude all possible physical causes before ascribing the agitation to the dementing process.

The most important cause of problem behaviors that must be excluded is pain. People with advanced dementia cannot articulate their pain or explain where the pain is located because of their impairment(s) of speech. They may not comprehend questions related to pain. Pain may be caused by multiple conditions, including urinary retention, fecal impaction, abdominal inflammation or obstruction, arthritis, or fractures. Fractures may occur even in people who are nonambulatory without evidence of fall or injury and require careful evaluation. Because the pain may be increased during the body movements that are required to provide care, fractures may also increase resistiveness.

Other medical conditions that may lead to agitation include shortness of breath caused by cardiovascular disease and chronic obstructive pulmonary disease. Increased anxiety and agitation also may be a side effect of pharmacotherapy (e.g., bronchodilators). The side effects of drugs may also induce sedation and apathy. Another common cause of behavior disorders is development of an infection. People with advanced dementia are at high risk for developing urinary tract infection and pneumonia (Volicer, 1996). The symptoms of these infections may be subtle because older adults may not develop increased body temperature. Sometimes the infection manifests itself only by a behavior change, nutritional change, or particular body posture. Metabolic disorders, including renal failure, dehydration, hyponatremia (i.e., a lower than normal concentration of sodium in the blood), hypo- or hyperglycemia (i.e., a lower or higher, respectively, concentration of glucose in the blood), hepatic failure, thyroid dysfunction, hypercalcemia (i.e., a higher than normal concentration of calcium in the blood), and anemia, also may affect the behavior of people with dementia. Another physical cause of altered behavior is sensory deprivation, which may cause a person's withdrawal or apathy.

PRIMARY AND SECONDARY CONSEQUENCES OF DEMENTIA

When all possible medical causes are excluded, the dementing process itself must be analyzed in order to initiate optimal management for problem behaviors. Progressive dementia has three main behavioral consequences: functional impairment, depression, and delusions/hallucinations (Volicer, Hurley, & Mahoney, 1997). These primary consequences cause by themselves or in combination secondary consequences, which include the inability to initiate meaningful activities, dependency in the activities of daily living (ADLs), anxiety, and spatial disorientation. Peripheral symptoms of dementia, such as agitation, apathy, and resistiveness, are caused by the primary and secondary consequences of progressive dementia and should not be treated in isolation. In the absence of disturbing hallucinations and depression, provision of meaningful activities is the most important management strategy. It was reported that distracting community-dwelling older adults with dementia using meaningful activities improved their mood during a dysphoric episode (Merriam, Aronson, Gaston, Wey, & Katz, 1988).

ENVIRONMENTAL FACTORS

In addition to physical factors, it is important to realize that a person's behavior represents an interaction between the person and his or her environment. Four environmental factors influence a person's behavior: caregiving strategies, social environment, physical environment, and medical treatment.

Caregivers must realize that they cannot change the behavior of people with dementia; they can change only their own behavior or environment. It is not possible for caregivers to impose their reality on people with dementia because these older adults are not able to reason rationally (Raia & Koenig-Coste, 1996). Therefore, caregivers must enter the reality of people with dementing illnesses and use "white lies," if necessary, to improve behavior or achieve their caregiving goals.

Caregivers should never say no because such a response may lead to a confrontation and escalation of behavior problems. They must use distraction or delaying tactics to prevent or stop care recipients' inappropriate behaviors. Although people with dementia may have difficulties communicating verbally, they are able to perceive and express emotions (Tappen, 1997). Caregivers must validate these emotions and maintain a cheerful and unhurried attitude when dealing with older adults with dementia.

The social environment involves the interactions among residents and among residents and visitors. Behavior problems frequently occur if residents with dementia reside in the same area as residents who are cognitively intact. Often, people with dementia enter the rooms of other residents and rummage through their belongings; occasionally, they may lie down on others' beds. Such behaviors are upsetting to residents who are cognitively intact, but are not problematic on a dementia-specific care unit (DSCU) because, often, residents with cognitive impairment do not remember which room is theirs. Similarly, it is easier to prevent elopement by securing the doors of the DSCU than by trying to intercept residents who leave the unit and trigger an alarm.

The level of noise, intensity of light, and physical layout are aspects of the physical environment that may affect a resident's behavior. A high noise level often triggers agitated behaviors. The intensity of light in most long-term care facilities is insufficient to ensure the synchronization of circadian rhythms (Satlin, Volicer, Stopa, & Harper, 1995; see also Chapter 8). It was reported that a higher light intensity promotes the body's secretion of melatonin, which is an important factor in the maintenance of regular sleep patterns (Hashimoto et al., 1997). Caregivers also must modify the environment to ensure care recipients' safety and to support recipients' remaining functional abilities.

Medical treatments may provoke or exacerbate behavior disorders. Often, individuals with dementia do not understand the need for diagnostic and therapeutic procedures and do not cooperate with them. Aggressive medical interventions require physical or chemical restraints to prevent the person with dementia from removing intravenous catheters and other medical devices. Therefore, the burden of a medical treatment must be compared with its benefit and the treatment modified according to the person's previous wishes or his or her best interests (Hurley, Bottino, & Volicer, 1994). The maintenance of the comfort of people with advanced dementia may be a more important consideration than ensuring survival at all costs (Volicer, 1993).

PSYCHOLOGICAL WELL-BEING

It is difficult to evaluate the degree of psychological well-being in individuals with advanced dementia, who, because of impaired speech, are unable to report their subjective states. However, these psychological states may be evaluated by observing the person's facial expression, vocalization characteristics, and body language. Such an observation allows discomfort in noncommunicative people with dementia to be rated (Hurley, Volicer, Hanrahan, Houde, & Volicer, 1992).

The evaluation of older adults who exhibited problem behaviors showed that different instruments measure psychological states that are, to a large extent, separate from each other. Based on these data the present authors proposed that psychological well-being can be evaluated by three scales that have the following end-points: happy–sad, engaged–apathetic, and calm–agitated (Volicer et al., manuscript in preparation). The optimal state of well-being is represented by a calm individual, happily engaged in a meaningful activity. This ideal may be difficult to achieve in all residents with dementia, but it should be a goal of behavior management strategies.

METHODS FOR INCREASING PSYCHOLOGICAL WELL-BEING

Multiple strategies have been developed for the management of behavioral consequences of advanced dementia (Table 1). The creation of a therapeutic environment underlies all of these interventions and is based on knowing the preferences, remaining abilities, and patterns of response of the person with dementia. In using environmental modifications one strives to maximize safety and autonomy and to avoid known triggers of behavioral symptoms. Some interventions are supported by research, whereas others are derived theoretically and await empirical support. Although methodological concerns, such as sampling and measurement issues, exist for many of the studies, they are included as the state-of-the-art and as a stimulus for further investigations. The interventions outlined in Table 1 are classified according to the category of evidence as follows: "A" indicates some research support, "B" represents expert opinion/clinical evidence/theory, "C" is empirical support from other populations, and "D" indicates review articles.

The authors describe in detail two novel interventions, simulated presence therapy and Snoezelen, that are especially suitable for people with moderate to severe dementia. These older adults experience short attention span and, often, are difficult to engage in a group setting. More research is needed to develop additional management strategies for such individuals.

SIMULATED PRESENCE THERAPY

People with dementia experience difficulty becoming engaged in meaningful activities, but many respond well to contact with family members or staff. However, the resources available do not allow one-to-one attention at all times when the individual is awake. Some residents respond well to radio or television, but very often these media do not provide optimal stimulation because the residents may experience comprehension difficulties and decreased attention span. Simulated presence therapy (SPT) is an effort to provide social contact for residents with dementia in a cost-effective manner.

Table 1. Selected behavioral interventions for the management of the behavioral consequences of advanced dementia

Behavior	Category of evidence	Intervention	Ref.
All	A/B/C	Behavior diary/behavior mapping; rationale Assessment of ABCs (Antecedents, Behaviors, Consequences) focuses care on key variables; provides a conceptual framework for interventions Provides baseline data for evaluation of therapeutic effectiveness of interventions Identification of change in behavior may signal physical illness, delirium, acute need Pattern identification targets timing of interventions Provides substrate for design of behavior modification by altering antecedents or consequences Acknowledges variability and complexity of behavior	Beck, Robinson, & Baldwin, 1992; Burgener, Jirovec, Murrell, & Barton, 1992; Burgener & Shimer, 1993; Burgio, Scilley, Davis, & Cadman, 1993; Cohen-Mansfield, Marx, & Rosenthal, 1989; Cohen-Mansfield & Werner, 1995; Corrigan, Yudofsky, & Silver, 1993; Gerdner & Buckwalter, 1994; Kolanowski et al., 1994; Ryden, Bossenmaier, & McLachlan, 1991; Yurick, Burgio, & Paton, 1995
	B	Individualized care	Haap, Williams, Strumpf, & Burger, 1996; Kayser-Jones, 1996; Vogelpohl, Beck, Heacock, & Mercer, 1996
	B	Try to understand behavior from perspective of person with dementia	Kovach & Meyer-Arnold, 1996; Rader, Lavelle, Hoeffer, & McKenzie, 1996
	A	Staff education/caregiver training	Rovner, Steele, Shmuely, & Folstein, 1996
	B	Geriatric mental health education and training programs by psychiatric/mental health nurses in long-term care	Smith et al., 1994

"Behavior disorder"	A	A.G.E. dementia care program: Activities, Guidelines for Psychotropic Medications, Educational rounds	Rovner, Steele, Shmuely, & Folstein, 1996
	A	Behavior analysis to provide systematic cues and reinforcements for desired behaviors	Boehm, Whall, Cosgrove, Locke, & Schlenk, 1995
	B	Development of internal nurse specialists	Smith, Mitchell, & Buckwalter, 1995
Agitation	A	Music Relaxing music during meals	Goddaer & Abraham, 1994 Ragneskog, Kihlgren, Karlsson, & Norberg, 1996
		Calming music	Tabloski, McKinnon-Howe, & Remington, 1995
		Favorite music Relaxation SPT	Casby & Holm, 1994 Synder, Egan, & Burns, 1995b Woods & Ashley, 1995
	A	Animal-assisted therapy	Zisselman, Rovner, Shmuely, & Ferrie, 1996
	B	Hand massage Physical contact, animal-assisted therapy, stimulus control, behavior modification, simple communication	Snyder, Egan, & Burns, 1995a Teri et al., 1992
	B	Treat pain and avoid restraints Minimize use of restraining devices	Cohen-Mansfield & Werner, 1995 Weinrich, Egbert, Eleazer, & Haddock, 1995
	B	Reduce noise level Snoezelen	Crowther & Volicer, unpublished observation

(continued)

Table 1—continued

Behavior	Category of evidence	Intervention	Ref.
ADL dependence	A	Support independence in dressing using levels of assistance, standard and problem-oriented strategies	Vogelpohl, Beck, Heacock, & Mercer, 1996
		Combined behavior management and mutual goal setting	Blair, 1995
	B	Prevention of excess disability	Beck, 1988; Beck, Heacock, Rapp, & Mercer, 1993; Burgener, Jirovec, Murrell, & Barton, 1992
		Compensate for losses while preserving remaining abilities	Kolanowski, 1995
		Feeding Behavior Inventory, to identify mealtime behaviors that interfere with self-feeding	Durnbaugh, Haley, & Roberts, 1996
		Interventions to promote functional feeding	Van Ort & Phillips, 1992, 1995
Aggression	A	Caregiver training using R.E.S.P.E.C.T. (Recognize/Empathize/Support/Prevent/Enhance/Care/Take time) model	Maxfield, Lewis, & Cannon, 1996
	B	Staff education on dementia and aggression	Hagen & Sayers, 1995
		Prevent or reduce aggression by avoiding known triggers; environmental stressors such as invasion of personal space, fatigue, fear, discomfort, loss of control	Ryden, Bossenmaier, & McLachlan, 1991
	B	Snoezelen	Brown, Jones, & Volicer, manuscript in preparation
	C/D	Token economy/aggression replacement/decelerative techniques	Corrigan, Yudofsky, & Silver, 1993

Category	Level	Intervention	Reference
Apathy	A	SPT	Woods & Ashley, 1995
	A	Video Respite	Lund, Hill, Caserta, & Wright, 1995
Depression	A	Reminiscence	Rentz, 1995
	A/B	Validation therapy	Bleathman & Morton, 1992; Kelly & Vanderslott, 1995; Morton & Bleathman, 1991
	B	Reminiscence and validation	Hall et al., 1995; Nugent, 1995
	A/C	Supportive and cognitive-behavioral psychotherapy beneficial in early stages of disease	Reifler et al., 1989
	A/B	Cognitive/behavioral interventions	Teri & Gallagher-Thompson, 1991
	A	Identifying pleasant activities	Teri & Logsdon, 1991
	A	Pleasant Events Schedule-AD and caregiver problem solving	Teri, Logsdon, Uomoto, & McCurry, 1997
	A/B/C/D	Clinical Practice Guideline	Depression Guideline Panel, 1993
	B	Unconditional positive regard	Hall & Buckwalter, 1987
Wandering	B	Environmental therapies: creating a structured activity schedule, placing lines on the floor	Holmberg, 1997; Teri et al., 1992
	D	Typology of wandering with associated assessments, interventions, and environmental modifications	Goldsmith, Hoeffer, & Rader, 1995; Hall et al., 1995
Anxiety	A	Reduction of environmental stress through DSCU structure, predictable routines, and continuity of care	Swanson, Maas, & Buckwalter, 1993
	A	Program of music, exercise, touch, and relaxation	Schwab, Rader, & Doan, 1985

(continued)

Table 1—*continued*

Behavior	Category of evidence	Intervention	Ref.
Anxiety—*continued*	B	Anticipate and prevent fear-producing stimuli; use a calm, gentle approach; maintain eye contact; explain all care; provide structured and predictable environment; use anxiety as a barometer for stress; as anxious behaviors occur, simplify stimuli; maintain consistency of personal and physical environments and routine	Hall & Buckwalter, 1987
Functional impairment Cognitive	A	Home-based active cognitive stimulation; maintain levels of cognitive and behavioral functioning (mild to moderate dementia of the Alzheimer's type)	Quayhagen, Quayhagen, Corbeil, Roth, & Rodgers, 1995
	A	Interpreting reality/maintaining normality/meeting basic needs/managing behavior disturbances	Rantz & McShane, 1995
	A	Validation therapy	Bleathman & Morton, 1992; Scanland & Emershaw, 1993
	A	Music as a memory trigger to improve communication	Sambandham & Schirm, 1995
	D	Standardized care plan of goals and interventions for managing a range of cognitive problems/needs	Hall et al., 1995
Physical	A	Walking program	Koroknay, Werner, Cohen-Mansfield, & Braun, 1995; MacRae et al., 1996
	B/C	Day treatment programs, structured activities, and respite services can prolong functioning of people with dementia in their home	Mace & Rabins, 1991

164

Delusions/ hallucinations	B/D	Distraction by involving resident in activity; respond to resident's feeling rather than argue or correct; monitor response to medications and side effects	Carlson, Fleming, Smith, & Evans, 1995
Resistiveness	A/B/D	Avoid precipitating factors: exaggerated startle response, modesty and attempts to maintain privacy, intrusion into personal space, desire to keep caregivers away, intense frustration	Potts, Richie, & Kass, 1996; Ryden, Bossenmaier, & McLachlan, 1991; Sloane et al., 1995
Spatial disorientation	B/D	Environmental modifications (half-doors, signs, visual aids)	Carlson, Fleming, Smith, & Evans, 1995
	A	Sensory integration	Robichaud, Hébert, & Desrosiers, 1994
	A	Alter feeding environment (context)	Phillips & Van Ort, 1993; Van Ort & Phillips, 1995
Food refusal		Use relaxing music to buffer noise level in dining rooms	Goddaer & Abraham, 1994
		Touch and verbal cueing	Lange-Alberts & Shott, 1994

165

SPT is based on the premise that dementia affects predominantly recent memory and that even people with moderate to severe dementia retain some long-term memory. This therapy utilizes these preserved memories to engage the individual in reminiscing, evoke positive emotions, and increase psychological well-being. SPT uses a personalized interactive audiotape that contains selected references that evoke preserved memories and positive emotions (Woods & Ashley, 1995). This tape is made by a family member or staff member ("caller") during a normal, spontaneous telephone conversation with the individual with dementia. Before the tape is made the family member is asked to complete a memory inventory form, which inquires about the topics he or she usually discusses with the resident during a visit and as to which of these topics evokes positive responses. These topics include best-loved people, important life events, family anecdotes, prayers, poems, hobbies, and interests (Woods & Ashley, 1995). The guidelines for the taped conversation concentrate on two or three themes repeated in various ways, and encourage communicating phrases of affection and conveying a positive emotion through nuances of voice as well as content. The tape is edited to preserve the "caller's" input with responses replaced by soundless spaces, which gives the resident the opportunity to respond to the input. The resulting one-sided personalized conversational audiotape is played for a resident by using a headset and a mobile autoreverse tape player enclosed in a hip pack. It is possible to play the 15- to 20-minute-long tape repeatedly because of the effects of dementia on short-term memory.

Efficacy of Simulated Presence Therapy

A feasibility study of SPT was conducted with 27 nursing facility residents who exhibited at least one of the following behaviors: "social isolation" (apathy), agitation, and "aggressive" behavior (resistiveness) (Woods & Ashley, 1995). Apathy was found most commonly, occurring in 93% of residents studied; agitation occurred in 67% and "aggression" in 7% of the residents. Of the 27 residents studied, 22 (81.5%) showed improvement with SPT. SPT was most effective in decreasing apathy (84% of residents responded) and less effective in decreasing agitation (78% of residents responded). In two residents who exhibited both apathy and agitation, SPT improved apathy but not agitation. Only two residents exhibited "aggression" and SPT improved this behavior in one of them.

An additional pilot study evaluated SPT in nine nursing facility residents. Disruptive behavior and social isolation were evaluated before the SPT trial and during a period of 2 months when SPT was administered twice a day. SPT significantly improved both disruptive behavior and social isolation when average scores for seven administrations were compared. When all observations were combined, SPT improved problem behavior 91% of the time. In 7% of the observations, the behavior either did not change or worsened, and SPT intervention was refused in 2% of the observations.

In a large multicenter trial involving 54 subjects, SPT was compared with a placebo (tape of newspaper reading) and "usual care" (one-to-one staff interaction) (Camberg et al., manuscript in preparation). Each study subject was exposed to all three conditions in random order for 3.5 weeks. According to nursing facility staff reports, SPT improved agitated behavior 75% more often than when a placebo was administered and 35% more often than when "usual care" was provided. When SPT was employed for withdrawn behavior, staff reported improvement at three times the frequency of placebo intervention and 80% more than when "usual care" was provided. In addition, ratings by trained independent observers, who were blind to the type of tape being used, showed that study subjects exposed to either SPT or "usual care" were more likely to display a happy facial expression than were those who were exposed to placebo. In this study SPT intervention was refused 3% of the time and placebo 5% of the time.

The results of all three studies indicate that SPT provides a strategy by which nursing facility residents can be engaged in pleasurable and personally meaningful activity using a minimum amount of staff time. SPT can be used as a substitute for one-to-one staff interaction when staff are involved in the care of other residents or as an addition to an existing activity program.

SNOEZELEN

One of the most difficult challenges in caring for people with severe cognitive impairment is finding appropriate leisure activities, particularly for older adults with dementia. The "normal" world is often confusing and threatening for people with profound or severe cognitive disabilities, and it is one that they find difficult to control, engage in, or understand. In general, they are controlled by other people, coerced into activities by others, or left in environments that may be nonstimulating.

Snoezelen ("Snooze-el-en") is a multisensory experience designed to gently stimulate the primary senses. This therapy springs from the belief that all human beings need stimulation and recreation, even people with special needs (Haggar & Hutchinson, 1991). The term Snoezelen (a trademark of ROMPA, Goyt Side Road, Chesterfield, England) is a Dutch contraction that means "to sniff and doze." The word arose from a desire to describe the comfortable, lazy feeling this therapeutic environment fosters. Snoezelen uses a combination of soft lighting effects, gentle music, tactile surfaces, and essential oils to stimulate the senses in a comfortable, safe environment (Figure 1). Snoezelen provides a wide range of sensory experiences that improve the quality of life for the individual with dementia. The greatest asset of Snoezelen lies in its ability to provide meaningful activity without requiring intellectual reasoning or verbal responses. This asset enables participants to engage at whatever level is appropriate for them, resulting in a release of stress and frustration.

Snoezelen is a means of stimulating the primary senses of sight, touch, hearing, and smell. Providing the Snoezelen environment (e.g., deciding which equip-

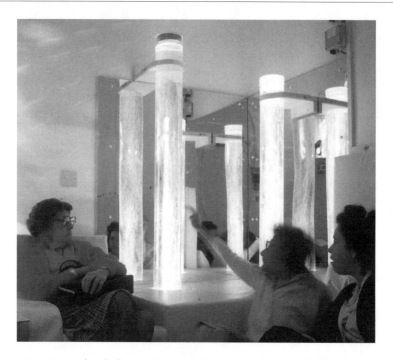

Figure 1.   Snoezelen helps to improve the quality of life of older people with Alzheimer's disease and related dementias. (Photograph courtesy of ROMPA® International, Chesterfield, England. sales@rompa.co.uk.)

ment to use, the layout of the room) has endless variations, but therein lies the success of Snoezelen—whether an entire suite or a few portable pieces of equipment are provided, Snoezelen is adaptable to the unique needs of each individual. The primary aims of Snoezelen are to

Provide a stimulating environment that heightens awareness

Provide an interesting atmosphere that encourages participants to explore their environment

Provide a secure environment, allowing participants mental and physical relaxation

Provide an unrestrained atmosphere in which participants feel able to enjoy themselves

Efficacy of Snoezelen

Snoezelen was developed originally for children with learning disabilities. The initial research involving older adults was conducted at the Kings Park Community Hospital in London and used a room containing a wide variety of equipment designed to provide sensory stimulation (Pinkney & Barker, 1994). The study investigated the effects of Snoezelen on mood and behavior, the most appropriate use of Snoezelen for older adults, and the role of staff during Snoezelen therapy. The recommendations that resulted from this study were to limit attendance to two residents and one staff member, which allows for ease of conversation and interaction. Gradually lowering or increasing the lighting within the room when initiating or concluding a session allowed individuals to remain relaxed. The study also found that staff roles needed to be adjusted because their approach to residents became that of enabler rather than provider of an activity.

The Keswick Multi-Care Center in Baltimore, Maryland, has developed a Snoezelen room for their residents with Alzheimer's disease. The goal was to soothe the fear, anxiety, and confusion often found in people with Alzheimer's disease. One report (Hendren, 1996) described the room this way: "A low glare light fills an 11 × 11 foot chamber with milk-white walls and furniture. A curtain of fiberoptic tubes changes colors, a wind machine blows gently, a glass water tower bubbles. A projector casts a stream of animated pictures on a wall, and the sounds of chimes mingled with songbirds waft through the room." The residents of Keswick were provided with 30 minutes of Snoezelen each week. Staff or family members accompanied residents and were able to introduce familiar smells, such as spices or perfumes, that help to spark positive memories and bring those memories to present consciousness. This type of "here-and-now" therapy helps to create a relaxing sensory environment for older adults, many of whom are struggling with an ever-diminishing sensory environment.

A portable Snoezelen program for people who are less ambulatory was developed at the Edith Nourse Rogers Memorial Veterans' Hospital in Bedford, Massachusetts (Figure 2). Two portable pieces of equipment were used: a specially designed audiotape of gentle music and a visual light display using a Solar 250 projector. The projector uses rotating wheels with colored oils to project moving colored shapes on a portable screen, a wall, or a ceiling.

Researchers have evaluated Snoezelen as an intervention for resistive behaviors in people with Alzheimer's disease (Brown, Jones, & Volicer, manuscript in preparation). This study evaluated the behavior of 29 older adults during 3 different treatment scenarios over 9 months. Dental hygiene treatment, which consisted of a toothbrush scrub, scaling, and fluoride treatment, was used as the constant stimulus for induction of resistive behavior. The control scenario consisted of dental hygiene care only. The second scenario began with 20 minutes of Snoezelen alone; then for the next 40 minutes, Snoezelen and dental hygiene treatment were provided simultaneously. The third scenario provided 60 minutes of Snoezelen alone followed by dental hygiene care. A Resistiveness to Care Scale (RTC-DAT; Mahoney et al., manuscript in preparation) was completed at the end of each treatment. (RTC-DAT is an observational scale that contains 13 items and rates behav-

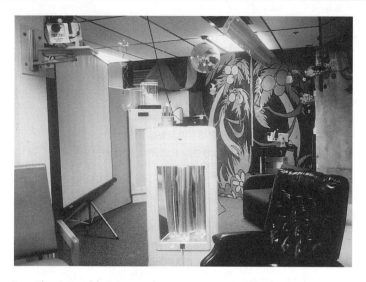

Figure 2.   The "portable" Snoezelen room at VA Bedford.

iors exhibited by people with dementia during care activities.) Although results fell slightly short of statistical significance the study did show a definite trend toward lower levels of resistiveness when Snoezelen was presented for 60 minutes prior to dental hygiene care. The highest level of resistiveness was observed with the two treatments together, possibly indicating overstimulation rather than relaxation.

Snoezelen also has been used at VA Bedford for patients with psychiatric disorders. Traditionally, nursing staff found morning care particularly difficult to provide because often patients would become loud, agitated, and aggressive. The portable components of Snoezelen were used on the psychiatric ward instead of transporting the patients to a Snoezelen room. Patients were gathered in a day room and Snoezelen was turned on. After approximately 20–30 minutes the nursing staff brought out patients to provide morning care and returned them to the day room when finished. Within a few days the patients began to anticipate the Snoezelen environment and would quiet down more easily and remain relatively calm during care.

CONCLUSION

Inability to initiate meaningful activity is one of the main causes of behavioral consequences of dementia. This inability is a result of functional impairment but may be aggravated by depression. Helping people with dementia to engage in meaningful activities decreases problem behaviors, such as agitation, repetitive vocalization, insomnia, and apathy. Also, meaningful activity may improve mood. Simulated presence therapy is a cost-effective strategy that provides meaningful activity for older adults with advanced dementia. Snoezelen can be used to provide either stimulation or a relaxing environment, which helps in managing the behavioral consequences of dementia.

REFERENCES

Beck, C. (1988). Measurement of dressing performance in persons with dementia. *American Journal of Alzheimer's Care and Related Disorders and Research, 3*(3), 21–25.

Beck, C., Heacock, P., Rapp, C.G., & Mercer, S.O. (1993). Assisting cognitively impaired elders with activities of daily living. *American Journal of Alzheimer's Care and Related Disorders and Research, 8*(6), 11–20.

Beck, C., Robinson, C., & Baldwin, B. (1992). Improving documentation of aggressive behavior in nursing home residents. *Journal of Gerontological Nursing, 18*(20), 21–24.

Blair, C.E. (1995). Combining behavior management and mutual goal setting to reduce physical dependency in nursing home residents. *Nursing Research, 44,* 160–165.

Bleathman, C., & Morton, I. (1992). Validation therapy with demented elderly. *Journal of Advanced Nursing, 13,* 511–514.

Boehm, S., Whall, A.L., Cosgrove, K.L., Locke, J.D., & Schlenk, E.A. (1995). Behavioral analysis and nursing interventions for reducing disruptive behaviors of patients with dementia. *Applied Nursing Research, 8,* 118–122.

Brown, E.J., Crowther, J., Jones, J.A., & Volicer, L. (manuscript in preparation). Snoezelen therapy as a means of reducing resistive behavior in Alzheimer's patients.

Burgener, S.C., Jirovec, M., Murrell, L., & Barton, D. (1992). Caregiver and environmental variables related to difficult behaviors in institutionalized demented elderly persons. *Journal of Gerontology, 47*(4), 242–249.

Burgener, S.C., & Shimer, R. (1993). Variables related to caregiver behaviors with cognitively impaired elders in institutional settings. *Research in Nursing & Health, 16,* 193–202.

Burgio, L.D., Scilley, K., Davis, P., & Cadman, S. (1993). Real-time behavioral observation of disruptive behaviors in the nursing home using laptop computers. *Gerontologist, 33,* 306.

Camberg, L., Hurley, A.C., Woods, P., Ooi, W.L., Ashley, J., Volicer, L., Odenheimer, G., & McIntyre, L.K. (manuscript in preparation). The use of audio recordings of selected memories to manage problem behaviors in Alzheimer's disease.

Carlson, D.L., Fleming, K.C., Smith, G.E., & Evans, J.M. (1995). Management of dementia-related behavioral disturbances: A nonpharmacologic approach. *Mayo Clinic Proceedings, 70,* 1108–1115.

Casby, J.A., & Holm, M.B. (1994). The effect of music on repetitive disruptive vocalizations of persons with dementia. *American Journal of Occupational Therapy, 48*(10), 883–889.

Chandler, J.D., & Chandler, J.E. (1988). The prevalence of neuropsychiatric disorders in a nursing home population. *Journal of Geriatric Psychiatry and Neurology, 1,* 71–76.

Cohen-Mansfield, J. (1988). Agitated behavior and cognitive functioning in nursing home residents: Preliminary results. *Clinical Gerontologist, 7*(3/4), 11–22.

Cohen-Mansfield, J., Marx, M.S., & Rosenthal, A.S. (1989). A description of agitation in a nursing home. *Journal of Gerontology: Medical Sciences, 44*(3), M77–M84.

Cohen-Mansfield, J., & Werner, P. (1995). Environmental influences on agitation: An integrative summary of an observational study. *American Journal of Alzheimer's Care and Related Disorders and Research, 10*(1), 32–39.

Corrigan, P.W., Yudofsky, S.C., & Silver, J.M. (1993). Pharmacological and behavioral treatments for aggressive psychiatric inpatients. *Hospital and Community Psychiatry, 44*(2), 125–133.

Depression Guideline Panel. (1993, April). *Depression in primary care: Volume 2. Treatment of major depression.* Clinical Practice Guideline No. 5. AHCPR Publication No. 93-0551. Rockville, MD: U.S. Department of Health and Human Services, Public Health Service, Agency for Health Care Policy and Research.

Durnbaugh, T., Haley, B., & Roberts, S. (1996). Assessing problem feeding behaviors in mid-stage Alzheimer's disease. *Geriatric Nursing, 17*(2), 63–67.

Gerdner, L.A., & Buckwalter, K.C. (1994). A nursing challenge: Assessment and management of agitation in Alzheimer's patients. *Journal of Gerontological Nursing, 20*(4), 11–20.

Goddaer, J., & Abraham, I.L. (1994). Effects of relaxing music on agitation during meals among nursing home residents with severe cognitive impairment. *Archives of Psychiatric Nursing, 8*(3), 150–158.

Goldsmith, S.M., Hoeffer, B., & Rader, J. (1995). Problematic wandering behavior in the cognitively impaired elderly. *Journal of Psychosocial Nursing, 33*(2), 6–12.

Haap, M.B., Williams, C.C., Strumpf, N.E., & Burger, S.G. (1996). Individualized care for frail elders: Theory and practice. *Journal of Gerontological Nursing, 22*(3), 6–14.

Hagen, B.F., & Sayers, D. (1995). When caring leaves bruises: The effects of staff education on resident aggression. *Journal of Gerontological Nursing, 21*(11), 7–16.

Haggar, L.E., & Hutchinson, R.B. (1991). Snoezelen: An approach to the provision of a leisure resource for people with profound and multiple handicaps. *Mental Handicap, 19*, 51–55.

Hall, G.R., & Buckwalter, K.C. (1987). Progressively lowered stress threshold: A conceptual model for care of adults with Alzheimer's disease. *Archives of Psychiatric Nursing, 1*, 349–406.

Hall, G.R., Buckwalter, K.C., Stolley, J.M., Gerdner, L.A., Garrand, L., Ridgeway, S., & Crump, S. (1995). Standardized care plan: Managing Alzheimer's patients at home. *Journal of Gerontological Nursing, 21*(1), 37–47.

Hashimoto, S., Kohsaka, M., Nakamura, K., Honma, H., Honma, S., & Honma, K. (1997). Midday exposure to bright light changes the circadian organization of plasma melatonin rhythm in humans. *Neuroscience Letters, 221*, 89–92.

Hendren, J. (1996). Baltimore's soothing room opens doors for Alzheimer's patients. *Maryland Maturity.*

Holmberg, S.K. (1997). Evaluation of a clinical intervention for wanderers on a geriatric nursing unit. *Archives of Psychiatric Nursing, 11*(1), 21–28.

Hurley, A.C., Bottino, R., & Volicer, L. (1994). Nursing role in advance proxy planning for Alzheimer patients. *Caring, 13*, 72–76.

Hurley, A., Odenheimer, G., Camberg, L., Woods, P., Ashley, J., & Volicer, L. (1995). Observation of agitated behaviors in patients with Alzheimer's disease. *Gerontologist, 35*, 161.

Hurley, A.C., Volicer, B.J., Hanrahan, P., Houde, S., & Volicer, L. (1992). Assessment of discomfort in advanced Alzheimer patients. *Research in Nursing & Health, 15*, 369–377.

Kayser-Jones, J. (1996). Mealtime in nursing homes: The importance of individualized care. *Journal of Gerontological Nursing, 22*(3), 26–31.

Kelly, J.S., & Vanderslott, J. (1995). Efficacy of validation therapy is unproven. *Professional Nurse, 10*(7), 408.

Knapp, M.J., Knopman, D.S., Solomon, P.R., Pendlebury, W.W., Davis, C.S., & Gracon, S.I. (1994). A 30-week randomized controlled trial of high-dose tacrine in patients with Alzheimer's disease. *Journal of the American Medical Association, 271*, 985–991.

Kolanowski, A.M. (1995). Disturbing behaviors in demented elders: A concept synthesis. *Archives of Psychiatric Nursing, 9*(4), 188–194.

Kolanowski, A., Hurwitz, S., Taylor, L.A., Evans, L., & Strumpf, N. (1994). Contextual factors associated with disturbing behaviors in institutionalized elders. *Nursing Research, 43*, 73–79.

Koroknay, V.J., Werner, P., Cohen-Mansfield, J., & Braun, J.V. (1995). Maintaining ambulation in the frail nursing home resident: A nursing administered walking program. *Journal of Gerontological Nursing, 21*(11), 18–24.

Kovach, C.R., & Meyer-Arnold, E.A. (1996). Coping with conflicting agendas: The bathing experience of cognitively impaired older adults. *Scholarly Inquiry for Nursing Practice, 10*(1), 23–42.

Lange-Alberts, M.E., & Shott, S. (1994). Nutritional intake: Use of touch and verbal cuing. *Journal of Gerontological Nursing, 20*(2), 36–40.

Lund, D.A., Hill, R.D., Caserta, M.S., & Wright, S.D. (1995). Video Respite: An innovative resource for family, professional caregivers, and persons with dementia. *Gerontologist, 35*, 683–687.

Mace, N.L., & Rabins, P.V. (1991). *The 36-hour day: A family guide to caring for persons with Alzheimer's disease, related dementing illness and memory loss in later life.* Baltimore: The Johns Hopkins University Press.

MacRae, P.D., Asplund, L.A., Schnelle, J.F., Ouslander, J.G., Abrahamse, A., & Morris, C. (1996). A walking program for nursing home residents: Effects on walk endurance, physical activity, mobility, and quality of life. *Journal of the American Geriatrics Society, 44*(2), 175–180.

Mahoney, E.K., Hurley, A.C., Volicer, L., Bell, M., Lane, P., Hartshorn, M., Rheume, Y., Gianotis, P., Lesperance, R., Novakoff, L., Sullivan, J., Timms, R., Warden, V., & McDonald, S. (1998). *Development and testing of the Resistiveness to Care Scale.* Manuscript submitted for publication.

Maxfield, M.C., Lewis, R.E., & Cannon, S. (1996). Training staff to prevent aggressive behavior of cognitively impaired elderly patients during bathing and grooming. *Journal of Gerontological Nursing, 22*(1), 37–43.

Merriam, A.E., Aronson, M.K., Gaston, P., Wey, S.-L., & Katz, I. (1988). The psychiatric symptoms of Alzheimer's disease. *Journal of the American Geriatrics Society, 36*, 7–12.

Morton, I., & Bleathman, C. (1991). The effectiveness of validation therapy in dementia: A pilot study. *International Journal of Geriatric Psychiatry, 6*, 327–330.

Nugent, E. (1995). Try to remember . . . Reminiscence as a nursing intervention. *Journal of Psychosocial Nursing and Mental Health Services, 33*(11), 7–11.

Paganini-Hill, A., & Henderson, V.W. (1996). Estrogen replacement therapy and risk of Alzheimer disease. *Archives of Internal Medicine, 156*, 2213–2217.

Phillips, L., & Van Ort, S. (1993). Measurement of mealtime interactions among persons with dementing disorders. *Journal of Nursing Measurement, 1*, 41–55.

Pinkney, L., & Barker, P. (1994). Snoezelen—An evaluation of a sensory environment used by people who are elderly and confused. In R. Hutchinson & J. Kewin (Eds.), *Sensations & disability.* Chesterfield, England: ROMPA.

Potts, H.W., Richie, M.F., & Kass, M.J. (1996). Resistance to care. *Journal of Gerontological Nursing, 22*(11), 11–16.

Quayhagen, M.P., Quayhagen, M., Corbeil, R.R., Roth, P.A., & Rodgers, J.A. (1995). A dyadic remediation program for care recipients with dementia. *Nursing Research, 44*, 153–159.

Rader, J., Lavelle, M., Hoeffer, B., & McKenzie, D. (1996). Maintaining cleanliness: An individualized approach. *Journal of Gerontological Nursing, 22*(3), 32–38.

Ragneskog, H., Kihlgren, M., Karlsson, I., & Norberg, A. (1996). Dinner music for demented patients: Analysis of video-recorded observations. *Clinical Nursing Research, 5*(3), 262–282.

Raia, P., & Koenig-Coste, J. (1996). Habilitation therapy: Realigning the planets. *Alzheimer's Association of Eastern Massachusetts Newsletter, 14*, 3–14.

Rantz, M.J., & McShane, R.E. (1995). Nursing interventions for chronically confused nursing home residents. *Geriatric Nursing, 16*, 22–27.

Reifler, B., Teri, L., Raskind, M., Veith, R., Barnes, R., While, E., & McLean, P. (1989). Double-blind trial of imipramine in Alzheimer's disease patients with and without depression. *American Journal of Psychiatry, 146*, 45–49.

Rentz, C.A. (1995). Reminiscence. A supportive intervention for the person with Alzheimer's disease. *Journal of Psychosocial Nursing and Mental Health Services, 33*(11), 15–20, 44–45.

Robichaud, L., Hébert, R., & Desrosiers, J. (1994). Efficacy of a sensory integration program on behaviors of inpatients with dementia. *American Journal of Occupational Therapy, 48*, 355–360.

Rogers, S.L., Friedhoff, L.T., Apter, J.T., Richter, R.W., Hartford, J.T., Walshe, T.M., Baumel, B., Linden, R.D., Kinney, F.C., Doody, R.S., Borison, R.L., & Ahem, G.L. (1996). The efficacy and safety of donepezil in patients with Alzheimer's disease: Results of a US multicentre, randomized, double-blind, placebo-controlled trial. *Dementia, 7*, 293–303.

Rovner, B.W., Kafonek, S., & Filipp, L. (1986). Prevalence of mental illness in a community nursing home. *American Journal of Psychiatry, 143*, 1446–1449.

Rovner, B.W., Steele, C.D., Shmuely, Y., & Folstein, M.F. (1996). A randomized trial of dementia care in nursing homes. *Journal of the American Geriatrics Society, 44*, 7–13.

Ryden, M.B., Bossenmaier, M., & McLachlan, C. (1991). Aggressive behavior in cognitively impaired nursing home residents. *Research in Nursing & Health, 14*, 87–95.

Ryden, M.B., & Feldt, K.S. (1992). Goal-directed care: Caring for aggressive nursing home residents with dementia. *Journal of Gerontological Nursing, 18*, 35–42.

Sambandham, M., & Schirm, V. (1995). Music as a nursing intervention for residents with Alzheimer's disease in long-term care. *Geriatric Nursing, 16*(2), 79–83.

Sano, M., Ernesto, C., Thomas, R.G., Klauber, M.R., Schafer, K., Grundman, M., Woodbury, P., Growdon, J., Cotman, D.W., Pfeiffer, E., Schneider, L.S., & Thal, L.J. (1997). A controlled trial of selegiline, alpha-tocopherol, or both as treatment for Alzheimer's disease. *New England Journal of Medicine, 336*, 1216–1222.

Satlin, A., Volicer, L., Stopa, E.G., & Harper, D. (1995). Circadian locomotor activity and core-body temperature rhythms in Alzheimer's disease. *Neurobiology of Aging, 16*, 765–771.

Scanland, S.G., & Emershaw, L.E. (1993). Reality orientation and validation therapy: Dementia, depression, and functional status. *Journal of Gerontological Nursing, 19*(6), 7–11.

Schwab, M., Rader, J., & Doan, J. (1985). Relieving the anxiety and fear in dementia. *Journal of Gerontological Nursing, 11*(5), 8–15.

Sloane, P.D., Rader, J., Barrick, A.-L., Hoeffer, B., Dwyer, S., McKenzie, D., Lavelle, M., Buckwalter, K., Arrington, L., & Pruitt, T. (1995). Bathing persons with dementia. *Gerontologist, 35*, 672–678.

Smith, M., Buckwalter, K.C., Garand, L., Mitchell, S., Albanese, M., & Kreiter, C. (1994). Evaluation of a geriatric mental health training program for nursing personnel in rural long-term care facilities. *Issues in Mental Health Nursing, 15*, 149–164.

Smith, M., Mitchell, S., & Buckwalter, K.C. (1995). Nurses helping nurses. Development of internal specialists in long-term care. *Journal of Psychosocial Nursing, 33*(4), 38–42.

Snyder, M., Egan, E.C., & Burns, K.R. (1995a). Efficacy of hand massage in decreasing agitation behaviors associated with care activities in persons with dementia. *Geriatric Nursing, 16*, 60–63.

Snyder, M., Egan, E.C., & Burns, K.R. (1995b). Interventions for decreasing agitation behaviors in persons with dementia. *Journal of Gerontological Nursing, 21*(7), 34–40.

Swanson, E.A., Maas, M.L., & Buckwalter, K.C. (1993). Catastrophic reactions and other behaviors of Alzheimer's residents: Special unit compared with traditional units. *Archives of Psychiatric Nursing, 7*, 277–283.

Tabloski, P.A., McKinnon-Howe, L., & Remington, R. (1995). Effects of calming music on the rest and activity disturbance in Alzheimer's disease. *American Journal of Alzheimer's Disease, 10*(1), 10–15.

Tappen, R.M. (1997). *Interventions for people with Alzheimer's disease: A caregiver's complete reference*. Baltimore: Health Professions Press.

Teri, L., & Gallagher-Thompson, D. (1991). Cognitive-behavioral interventions for treatment of depression in Alzheimer's patients. *Gerontologist, 31*, 413–416.

Teri, L., & Logsdon, R.G. (1991). Identifying pleasant activities for Alzheimer's disease patients: The Pleasant Events Schedule-AD. *Gerontologist, 31*(1), 124–127.

Teri, L., Logsdon, R.G., Uomoto, J., & McCurry, S.M. (1997). Behavioral treatment of depression in dementia patients: A controlled clinical trial. *Journal of Gerontology: Psychological Sciences, 52B*(4), P159–P166.

Teri, L., Rabins, P., Whitehouse, P., Berg, L., Reisberg, B., Sunderland, T., Eichelman, B., & Phillips, C. (1992). Management of behavior disturbance in Alzheimer disease: Current knowledge and future directions. *Alzheimer's Disease and Associated Disorders, 6*(2), 77–88.

Van Ort, S., & Phillips, L. (1992). Feeding nursing home residents with Alzheimer's disease. *Geriatric Nursing, 13*, 249–253.

Van Ort, S., & Phillips, L.R. (1995). Nursing interventions to promote functional feeding. *Journal of Gerontological Nursing, 21*(10), 6–14.

Vogelpohl, R.S., Beck, C.K., Heacock, P., & Mercer, S.O. (1996). "I can do it." Dressing: Promoting independence through individualized strategies. *Journal of Gerontological Nursing, 22*(3), 39–42.

Volicer, L. (1993). Alzheimer's disease: Course, management, and the hospice approach. *Nursing Home Medicine, 1*(5), 31–37.

Volicer, L. (1996). Clinical issues in advanced dementia. In S.B. Hoffman & M. Kaplan (Eds.), *Special care programs for people with dementia* (pp. 61–77). Baltimore: Health Professions Press.

Volicer, L., Camberg, L., Ashley, J., Woods, P., Hurley, A.C., Ooi, W.L., & McIntyre, K. (manuscript in preparation). Dimensions of psychological well-being in advanced dementia.

Volicer, L., Hurley, A.C., & Mahoney, E. (1997). Psychopharmacology and late-stage dementia behaviors. In C.R. Kovach (Ed.), *Late-stage dementia care: A basic guide* (pp. 143–155). Bristol, PA: Taylor & Francis.

Weinrich, S., Egbert, C., Eleazer, G.P., & Haddock, K.S. (1995). Agitation: Measurement, management, and intervention research. *Archives of Psychiatric Nursing, 9*(5), 251–260.

Woods, P., & Ashley, J. (1995). Simulated presence therapy: Using selected memories to manage problem behaviors in Alzheimer's disease patients. *Geriatric Nursing, 16*, 9–14.

Yurick, A., Burgio, L., & Paton, S.M. (1995). Assessing behaviors of nursing home residents: Use of microcomputer technology to promote objectivity in planning nursing interventions. *Journal of Gerontological Nursing, 21*(4), 29–34.

Zisselman, M.H., Rovner, B.W., Shmuely, Y., & Ferrie, P. (1996). A pet therapy intervention with geriatric psychiatry inpatients. *American Journal of Occupational Therapy, 50*(1), 47–51.

12

Pharmacological Treatment of Dementia and Behavior Disorders in Dementia

Rajeev Trehan, M.B.B.S., M.D., M.P.H.

Psychoactive medications are useful in the management of symptoms associated with dementia. However, their use must be approached with caution because older adults, who constitute the majority of people with dementia, experience diminished renal clearance, slowed hepatic metabolism, and diminished body mass. Smaller starting doses with smaller increments and longer intervals between increments are advisable. General medical conditions and other medicines may alter the fate of these agents further. In addition, older adults and people with dementia are more sensitive to side effects than are people who are younger and who do not have dementia.

The medications used in the treatment of dementia can be divided into two broad categories: for the treatment of dementia and for the treatment of behavior disturbances associated with dementia. Certainly, drugs may be effective in more than one domain. The treatment of people with dementia with combination regimens is not yet fully accepted, although such strategies are well established in the treatment of infectious diseases, depression, and other conditions. For example, the combination of a cholinesterase inhibitor and a selective serotonin reuptake inhibitor (SSRI; drugs used often in the treatment of depression) could be beneficial in the management of dementia. The addition of an antioxidant (e.g., vitamin E) to these inhibitors continues to be promising as an effective intervention (Sunderland et al., 1992).

TREATMENT OF DEMENTIA

Two of the most common types of dementia, Alzheimer's disease and vascular dementia, command the greatest attention among researchers in pharmacological interventions.

ALZHEIMER'S DISEASE

Various pharmacological approaches have been considered in the treatment of Alzheimer's disease. Among these are anti-inflammatory approaches; attempts to reduce beta-amyloid formation; interventions to reduce hyperphosphorylated tau protein; and attempts to improve cholinergic function, decrease cholinergic atrophy, and reduce oxidative damage (Schneider, 1996; Schneider & Tariot, 1994).

ANTI-INFLAMMATORY AGENTS

Considerable evidence supports the hypothesis that the inflammatory and immune systems are linked to the destruction of brain tissue associated with dementia (Aisen & Davis, 1994). Because they are well-known mediators of inflammatory and immune responses, cytokines such as interleukin-1 and interleukin-6 promote the synthesis of amyloid precursor protein (i.e., a normal brain protein that may have perfectly innocent functions, but is a necessary precursor of amyloid; amyloid is an insoluble protein found in plaques in the brains of people with Alzheimer's disease), which then may be processed (enzymatic proteins are involved in the formation of amyloid from the precursor) and transformed into potentially neurotoxic beta-amyloid. The role of nonsteroidal anti-inflammatory drugs (NSAIDs) in the body is a protective one, which is supported by evidence of an unexpectedly low prevalence of Alzheimer's disease in people with rheumatoid arthritis (Rogers et al., 1993). The NSAID indomethacin has been shown to stabilize cognitive function in people with Alzheimer's disease (Rogers et al., 1993). Aspirin in different daily doses has been credited for positive neuroprotective effects (Stewart, Kawas, Corrada, & Metter, 1997). A long-term trial using low-dose prednisone (10 mg/day) is under way, the hypothesis being that the known anti-inflammatory properties of prednisone should slow or prevent Alzheimer's disease (National Institute on Aging, 1997).

CHOLINERGIC AGENTS

The treatment of cognition with cholinergic agents (i.e., medicines that enhance acetylcholine, one of the main chemical messengers in the brain) has been the most promising and frequently used intervention for the cognitive decline experienced by people with Alzheimer's disease. Both muscarinic and nicotinic (i.e., the two types of receptors through which acetylcholine acts in the brain) cholinergic agonists have been considered. Some of the agents that have been used are xanomeline, milameline, SB202026, AF102B, and ABD418, most of which are in the early stages of development.

Cholinesterase inhibitors (CHEIs) are another large class of medicines that have been useful in treating dementia. CHEIs can be divided roughly into first- and second-generation agents. The first-generation agents are nonspecific in their inhibition of acetylcholinesterase, butyrylcholinesterase, and other peripheral cholinesterases (i.e., normally occurring enzymes that break down acetylcholine and other, similar neurochemicals). These agents include physostigmine, sustained-release physostigmine (Synapton SR), and tacrine. The second-generation CHEIs are longer acting, more predictable in their kinetics, and provide higher concentrations in the nervous system. They are more selective in their inhibition of cholinesterase and have fewer peripheral side effects than first-generation agents. Among the agents that belong to the second generation of CHEIs are donepezil, ENA 713 (Exelon), metrifonate, galanthamine, and eptastigmine. Of these, ENA 713 is a pseudoirreversible carbamate-selective cholinesterase inhibitor that is not metabolized by the hepatic microsomal system (Anand, Gharabawi, & Enz, 1996). The evidence that the benefits of CHEIs do not derive solely from an increase of acetylcholine in the clefts is mounting (Knopman et al., 1996). Neuroprotective action may come through the nicotinic receptors or neuroregenerative action through muscarinic receptor stimulation. Several of the first- and second-generation agents are examined in the following sections.

Tacrine hydrochloride (Cognex) is a centrally and peripherally acting, reversible, acridine-based CHEI potassium channel blocker, having an action of 4–6 hours and leading to nonspecific cholinesterase inhibition and increased amounts of intrasynaptic acetylcholine. It has good central nervous system penetration and a wide therapeutic range—80–160 mg/day, which is administered in four doses. The dosage must be increased gradually. Tacrine has been shown to lead to modest improvements in cognition in a substantial minority of older adults. However, up to 30% of older adults cannot tolerate this medicine because of the side effects of nausea and vomiting or liver damage (Clark & Arnold, 1997; Knapp et al., 1994). Greater improvement is found in older people with moderate cognitive impairment, and modest clinical evidence of neuroprotection also was found. After a 2-year follow-up, there was a delay in nursing facility placement and longer survival, more so with a higher dosage (Knopman et al., 1996). As mentioned, side effects are a problem with tacrine, particularly liver damage caused by transaminase elevation, which occurs in about 30% of patients. The elevation in liver transaminases is almost three times greater than normal and manifests in individuals within the first 12 weeks of treatment at a 40–80 mg/day dose. In addition, there are gastrointestinal side effects such as nausea, vomiting, and diarrhea, and some cholinergic side effects including bradycardia (i.e., a potentially dangerous slowing of the heart).

Donepezil hydrochloride (Aricept) also has been shown to lead to modest improvements in a substantial minority of older adults. This medication is a second-generation, piperazine-based, highly specific, reversible inhibitor of brain acetylcholinesterase. Because of its specificity donepezil has far fewer side effects—nausea, vomiting, and anorexia—than tacrine. Unlike tacrine, it has linear kinetics (i.e., the drug levels in the body are dictated in a relatively straightforward way with the doses taken) with dose predictability and more steady plasma levels. It has a long half-life of approximately 70 hours, which allows once-a-day dosing (the usual dose is 3–10 mg/day). A dose of 5 mg/day resulted in significantly improved quality of life and cognitive improvement in people with Alzheimer's disease (Rogers, Friedhoff, & the Donepezil Study Group, 1996).

Metrifonate is a prodrug that is converted to dichlorvos, an organophosphate with a long duration of action and essential irreversibility of cholinesterase inhibition in the central nervous system. It has been used to treat schistosomiasis. Metrifonate has a considerable blood–brain barrier and is rapidly metabolized, which together prevent high concentrations from gathering in the central nervous system. Improvements in cognitive function were seen in individuals receiving a weekly dose of 5 mg/kg (Becker, Colliver, & Elble, 1990).

NEUROPROTECTIVE AGENTS

Among the neuroprotective agents that are being used or studied for their efficacy in treating Alzheimer's disease are antioxidants, monoamine oxidase (MAO) inhibitors, vitamin E, ascorbic acid, coenzyme Q, idebenone, and nimodipine.

Because oxidative mechanisms may play a role in the loss of some neurons, the use of antioxidants in treating dementia is interesting. The aging brain is susceptible to oxidative stress, which can result in a neurodegenerative cascade involving disruption of DNA, damage to cell membranes, and neuronal death (LeBel & Bondy, 1991).

Selegiline (Eldepryl) is a selective type B MAO inhibitor that reduces the concentration of free radicals and neurotoxins. It can be administered in doses of 5–10 mg/day. A single large, well-conducted trial showed a significant delay in poor outcome during a 2-year period. However, it is associated with orthostatic hypotension (i.e., dizziness on rising from a sitting position), activation, and the risk of drug interactions (Sano et al., in press).

A single, large, well-conducted trial using vitamin E showed a significant delay in poor outcome (i.e., the inexorable poor prognosis of Alzheimer's disease was slowed slightly) during a 2-year period. A twice-daily dosage of 1,000 International Units is recommended. In vitamin K-deficient individuals, a smaller dosage of vitamin E must be used (Sano et al., in press).

OTHER AGENTS

Other agents that may be useful in treating Alzheimer's disease are nerve growth factor, estrogen, melatonin, and botanical and chelating agents. Nerve growth factor may be effective in slowing neuronal loss (Schneider, 1996). Estrogen supplementation has been shown to be beneficial in treating Alzheimer's disease, particularly in postmenopausal women (Sherwin, 1994). Melatonin is receiving increasing attention for its effects on the central nervous system. Botanical agents such as gingko biloba are being investigated for their protective properties, and chelating agents such as desferioxamine may be useful, but may be toxic and are not recommended (American Psychiatric Association, 1997).

VASCULAR DEMENTIAS

Vascular dementias are believed to be caused by the interruption of blood supply to the brain cells. The causes include sudden blockage of blood vessels by blood-borne plaques or emboli and gradual occlusions by atherosclerosis or other diseases. If neuronal death can be delayed, sometimes blood supply resumes and the cells may survive. At times, lack of blood supply leads to swelling (i.e., cerebral edema), which further impairs blood supply. If lack of blood supply can be prevented, the chance of neuronal survival may improve. Certain drugs may be useful or harmful at different times in the pathogenesis of vascular dementia.

MIXTURE OF ERGOT MESYLATES (HYDERGINE)

Ergot compounds are not recommended for the routine treatment of cognitive symptoms, but they may aid in the treatment of vascular dementias. Inconsistent findings in 150 studies over 40 years have failed to produce a consensus. A meta-analysis suggests a lack of statistically significant effects, but the findings for vascular dementia are somewhat more compelling (Schneider & Olin, 1994). A dose of 3 mg/day, which may be increased to 9 mg/day, has been used and produces only minor side effects, such as mild nausea and gastrointestinal distress. Hydergine is, however, contraindicated in people with psychosis.

DRUGS THAT DELAY NEURONAL DEATH

Several drugs—calcium channel blockers, free-radical scavengers, and adenosine analogs—are advocated for their ability to delay neuronal death in people with vascular dementia. Calcium channel blockers such as nimodipine in doses of 120 mg/day are favored, especially if the treatment is initiated within hours of the occurrence of stroke. A role in delaying the death of neurons has been suggested for free-radical scavengers such as allopurinol, vitamin E, and cytidine-5-diphosphocholine. Adenosine analogs such as cyclohexyladenosine also are thought to delay neuronal death.

DRUGS THAT REDUCE CEREBRAL EDEMA

Agents that aid in the reduction of cerebral edema include exogenous gangliosides, free-radical scavengers (e.g., MCI 186), and 21 amino steroids.

OTHER DRUGS

Diaschisis is the functional suppression of regions of the brain that are distant from the site of a primary injury and may have a role in dementia. Among the agents that are suggested to reduce diaschisis are amphetamines, alpha$_2$ agonists (e.g., yohimbine), alpha$_1$ receptor antagonists (e.g., phenoxybenzamine, prazosin), bromocriptine, and apomorphine.

Agents that reduce lipoproteinemia (i.e., lipoproteinemia indicates an excessive amount of blood-borne lipids in combination with carrier proteins; lipid deposits in the blood vessels could lead to blockages that may cause vascular dementias) have been justified as possible preventive measures against vascular pathology. Antiplatelet agents (Alexopoulos, 1996) have been used in stroke prevention because these agents tend to inhibit platelets from forming clumps and are believed to assist blood supply to at-risk areas of the circulation.

TREATMENT OF BEHAVIOR
DISTURBANCES ASSOCIATED WITH DEMENTIA

Behavior disturbances are common in people with dementia. The classification of these disturbances into classes of behaviors (e.g., agitation, psychosis, depression, insomnia) provides a useful guide to pharmacotherapeutic treatments for the behaviors.

AGITATION AND AGGRESSION

Antipsychotic agents, anticonvulsants, anxiolytics, antidepressants, cholinergic agents, hormones, lithium carbonate, and beta blockers are effective in the treatment of agitation and aggression associated with dementia.

Antipsychotic agents are best documented pharmacologically for the treatment of agitation in dementia. Their effects are modest but consistent and reliable. No single antipsychotic agent is better than another, and small doses are recommended. These agents are most useful in older adults with a psychotic component (Schneider, Pollock, & Lyness, 1990).

Anticonvulsants such as carbamazepine and valproic acid are used in treating agitation in people with dementia. The reports on the efficacy of carbamazepine from two double-blind, placebo-controlled, crossover studies (Tariot et al., 1994) conflict. It has been suggested that carbamazepine may be effective when blood serum levels of 8–12 µg/ml are achieved (Tariot et al., 1994). The side effects of carbamazepine are ataxia (i.e., unsteady gait), sedation, confusion, hyponatremia (i.e., a low level of sodium in the blood), and, rarely, bone marrow suppression.

The preliminary reports on the use of valproic acid and its enteric-coated derivative in reducing agitation in people with dementia are encouraging (Lott, McElroy, & Keys, 1995). Older adults who are physically and verbally aggressive and restless seem to respond best to this medication. The side effects of valproic acid include gastrointestinal disturbances, ataxia, hepatic toxicity, and, rarely, bone marrow suppression. A divided dose of 10 mg/kg/day in order to maintain serum levels between 50–100 µg/ml is recommended (Sival et al., 1994).

Anxiolytics are medicines that tend to reduce anxiety and have an overall calming effect. Benzodiazepines are used widely, but have not been well studied in people with dementia. They seem to perform better than placebos, but not as well as do antipsychotics. It is unfortunate that many observations are based on longer-acting agents in high doses, whereas it is well known that these agents are not preferred in older adults and many excellent, shorter-acting agents have long been available. The side effects of benzodiazepines include sedation, ataxia, paradoxic agitation (i.e., a phenomenon in which a medicine with an expected calming effect causes an exacerbation of agitated behavior), amnesia, tolerance, and withdrawal (Yeager, Farnett, & Ruzicka, 1995). Of the benzodiazepines, lorazepam and oxazepam are preferred for use in older people because these drugs do not require oxidative metabolism in the liver and do not produce active metabolites. Temazepam possesses characteristics similar to those of lorazepam and oxazepam, but it has a somewhat longer half-life; clonazepam has a much longer half-life. The suggested dosages of lorazepam are 0.5–1 mg every 6 hours; the suggested dosages of oxazepam are 7.5–15 mg one to four times every day (Hyman & Arana, 1987).

Another anxiolytic, buspirone hydrochloride, is prescribed generally for anxiety disorders. A modest amount of evidence exists that this 5-HT agonist may be effective at a dosage of 15–60 mg/day, with minimal side effects consisting mainly of headache, nervousness, and dizziness. It should be used with caution, if at all, in combination with SSRIs because of the possibility of precipitating a serotonin syndrome (Herrmann & Eryavec, 1993). In addition, individuals with severe hepatic or renal impairment should not take this medication. Low-dose buspirone was comparable in effectiveness to low-dose haloperidol, a tranquilizer used in treating psychotic disorders, in improving behavior in one study (Cantillon et al., 1996).

The use of antidepressants and mood stabilizers in treating agitation in older people with dementia has met with great success. Three such antidepressants are trazodone, sertraline, and citalopram. Trazodone, used in doses of 25–250 mg/day, in one dose or in divided doses, has been associated with improvement in agitated and aggressive behaviors in more than half of the older adults studied (Lebert, Pasquier, & Petit, 1994). Antidepressant side effects include postural hypotension, sedation, and dry mouth. Trazodone was compared with haloperidol in a double-blind, uncontrolled study, and both were effective. Trazodone was more successful than haloperidol in reducing repetitive behavior, verbal aggression, negativism, and resistance to care. Also, one third fewer individuals dropped out of the study due to adverse effects (Sultzer et al., 1997). Sertraline is a type B MAO inhibitor. At doses of 10 mg/day, individuals with dementia showed significant improvement in anxiety, depression, tension, and excitement scores on the Brief Psychiatric Rating Scale in a double-blind, placebo-controlled study (Tariot et al., 1987). Used primarily in people with bipolar disorder, lithium carbonate has been used in older adults with dementia exhibiting behavior problems because it is an effective mood stabilizer (Leibovici & Tariot, 1988). Citalopram, administered in doses of 20–30 mg/day, resulted in reduced confusion, irritability, and restlessness in people with Alzheimer's disease. Few side effects were noted (Nyth & Gottfries, 1990).

Cholinergic agents such as physostigmine, arecoline, nicotine, and tacrine have been reported to exert beneficial effects on behavioral disturbances in people with dementia, perhaps by improving cognitive function or cholinergic tone (Kanfer et al., 1996).

Hormones, such as estrogen and medroxyprogesterone acetate, have been shown to reduce physical aggression, including sexually inappropriate behaviors in older adult men (Kyomen, Nobel, & Wei, 1991). Beta blockers, namely propranolol, metoprolol, and pindolol, are effective in some older adults, but most respondents had unusual comorbidities, and large doses (e.g., as high as 200–300 mg/day of propranolol) were needed, which have the added risk of bradycardia, hypotension, and delirium.

PSYCHOSIS

Antipsychotics are the only documented pharmacological treatment for psychosis in people with dementia. No evidence of a difference in efficacy among antipsychotic agents has been documented. Because a number of potentially serious side effects occur (e.g., sedation, worsening of cognition), these medications must be used at the lowest effective dose. Adverse events, such as tardive dyskinesia (i.e., a relatively persistent involuntary movement, often of the mouth and tongue), for which older adults, women, and individuals with dementia are at greater risk, and neuroleptic malignant syndrome (i.e., a potentially lethal condition of high fever and muscular rigidity sometimes seen in patients taking antipsychotics), must be kept in mind. Some of the antipsychotics used in older adults are haloperidol, thioridazine, clozapine, risperidone, olanzapine, sertindole, depot antipsychotics, and physostigmine.

Haloperidol is the most widely used antipsychotic in older adults, and, as previously mentioned, its efficacy is probably offset by its potential for side effects (Reisberg et al., 1987). Thioridazine is a neuroleptic (i.e., drug that induces a state of quiescence, reduced motor activity, anxiety, indifference to surroundings). The side effect profile for thioridazine is concerned mainly with cardiovascular symptoms, but there are other side effects such as akathisia, parkinsonism, and tardive dyskinesia (Tune, Steel, & Cooper, 1991).

Clozapine is a novel antipsychotic that is thought to act on the limbic dopaminergic receptors, with low affinity for the striatum. Reports of experience with this agent present a mixed picture of efficacy and side effects. Certainly, there are fewer incidents of extrapyramidal syndromes, tardive dyskinesia, and neuroleptic malignant syndrome, but somewhat more sedation, hypotension, and risk of seizure (Salzman et al., 1995).

Risperidone is a benzisoxazole derivative with potent serotonin and dopamine receptor–blocking properties. Risperidone shows promise in its ability to reduce psychotic symptoms with less extrapyramidal features (Reyntgens et al., 1988), but the literature is confusing on the effectiveness of risperidone; the drug has been in common use only since the mid-1990s (Madusoodanan, Brenner, Araujo, & Abaza, 1995). Olanzapine is receiving attention for its excellent antipsychotic action with relatively few side effects, and sertindole is a new antipsychotic agent whose usefulness in reducing behavior problems in people with dementia holds promise. In doses of 1.25–3.75 mg/month, fluphenazine decanoate (Prolixin), a depot antipsychotic, has been known to reduce behavior disturbances in people with dementia (Gottlieb et al., 1988). The drug is long acting, and the side effects for older adults include development of tardive dyskinesia. Physostigmine was found to decrease delusional symptoms in a trial studying people with Alzheimer's disease (Cummings et al., 1993).

DEPRESSION

Depression is a significant problem in people with dementia, particularly older adults. In assessing the efficacy of a particularly pharmacological intervention, one must bear in mind that placebo responses occur frequently in people with dementia who have wide fluctuations in their mood. Early improvements should be viewed as possible fluctuations. The medications commonly used in the treatment of older adults with dementia who are depressed include SSRIs, trazodone, tricyclic antidepressants, bupropion, venlafaxine, maprotiline, psychostimulants, bromocriptine, and amantadine.

SSRIs are the first-line treatments for depression in people with dementia despite their associated side effects. Some of the side effects associated with SSRIs include nausea and vomiting, agitation, akathisia, parkinsonism, sexual dysfunction, and weight loss. Fluoxetine, 5–10 mg/day, can be increased at several-week intervals to a maximum dose of 40–60 mg/day. Paroxetine, 5–10 mg/day, with increases at 1- to 2-week intervals up to 40 mg/day, is useful. Sertraline at a starting dose of 25 mg/day and increases at 1- to 2-week intervals up to 150–200 mg/day is recommended. Citalopram proved to be more effective than placebo on the

Hamilton Depression Scale, the Clinical Global Impression, the Montgomery Asberg Depression Rating Scale, and the Gottfries-Brane-Steen scale (Nyth et al., 1992).

Trazodone, 25–50 mg/day, with weekly increases up to 300–400 mg/day, is a fairly safe and effective antidepressant in older adults. One side effect to watch for is sedating action. Bupropion, which can be initiated at 37.5 mg twice a day with weekly increases of up to the 350–450 mg/day range in divided doses, is an effective antidepressant with some risk of seizures at high doses. No dose should exceed 150 mg.

When administering tricyclic antidepressants, a secondary amine such as nortriptyline is useful starting at 10–25 mg/day, increasing weekly to 100–150 mg/day, and titrating to blood levels of 60–125 ng/ml. Desipramine, 25–50 mg/day, with weekly increases of up to 200 mg/day and blood levels up to 120 ng/ml, is quite effective. Some of the side effects of desipramine include hypotension, cardiac conduction delay, cholinergic side effects, sedation, confusion, and delirium (Reifler et al., 1989).

Venlafaxine can be initiated at 18.75–37.5 mg twice a day, with weekly increases reaching a dosage range of 300–375 mg/day. However, this medication is associated with an elevation in blood pressure. If the antidepressant response is encouraging, antihypertensives may be used to decrease blood pressure. Maprotiline is a sedating and slightly anticholinergic agent. No study to date has proved its efficacy in reducing depression in older adults (Fuchs et al., 1993).

Psychostimulants such as D-amphetamine and methylphenidate are particularly useful in apathetic individuals. The side effect profile of psychostimulants includes tachycardia, restlessness, agitation, sleep disturbances, and appetite suppression. A dose of 2.5–5 mg every morning, increased every 3 days up to a dosage range of 30–40 mg/day, may be administered.

Bromocriptine can be initiated at 1.25 mg twice a day and increased up to 2.5 mg twice a day in apathetic people with dementia. The drug carries with it a risk of psychosis, confusion, and dyskinesias. Amantadine can be used in doses of 100–200 mg/day, but it may have some cholinergic side effects such as delirium.

INSOMNIA

Sleep disorders can lead to disruptive behaviors in older adults with dementia. Some of the drugs used to treat insomnia are zolpidem, trazodone, antipsychotics, melatonin, nortriptyline, benzodiazepines, and chloralhydrate.

Zolpidem, 10 mg/day, has been proved to be superior to placebo in multiple sleep outcome studies (Shaw, Curson, & Coquetin, 1992). Trazodone, 25–100 mg at bedtime, may be used to help older individuals sleep (Satlin, 1994). Antipsychotics in low doses, such as haldol at 0.5–1 mg, are useful in the management of sleep problems in people with dementia. Similarly, thioridazine may be effective because of its relatively greater sedating action. Preliminary evidence holds that the hormone melatonin may be beneficial in the treatment of sleep disturbances in older individuals (Singer et al., 1995). Nortriptyline given at bedtime in doses of 25–50 mg has been used for its sleep-inducing properties. Benzodiazepines and chloralhydrate usually are not recommended for long-term use because of the risk of daytime sedation, tolerance, rebound insomnia, worsening cognition, disinhibition, and delirium. If necessary, lorazepam at 0.5–1 mg and oxazepam at 7.5–15 mg may be administered at bedtime.

CONCLUSION

The list of medications that are useful in the treatment of dementia is growing. In the next few decades we will see the introduction of many drugs designed to protect the brain from the effects of degeneration. At the same time, there will be continued improvements in the agents available to treat behavior disturbances, such as agitation, psychosis, depression, and insomnia, as they relate to dementia.

REFERENCES

Aisen, P.S., & Davis, K.L. (1994). Inflammatory mechanisms in Alzheimer's disease: Implications for therapy. *American Journal of Psychiatry, 151,* 1105–1113.

Alexopoulos, G.S. (1996). The treatment of depressed, demented patients. *Journal of Clinical Psychiatry, 57*(Suppl. 14), 14–20.

American Psychiatric Association. (1997). Practice guidelines for the treatment of patients with Alzheimer's disease and other dementias of late life. *American Journal of Psychiatry, 154*(Suppl. 5), 1–39.

Anand, R., Gharabawi, G., & Enz, A. (1996). Efficacy and safety results of the early phase studies with Exelon (ENA 713) in Alzheimer's disease: An overview. *Journal of Drug Development and Clinical Practice, 8,* 109–116.

Becker, R.E., Colliver, J., & Elble, R. (1990). Effects of metrifonate, a long-acting cholinesterase inhibitor in Alzheimer's disease: Report of an open trial. *Drug Development Research, 19,* 425–434.

Cantillon, M., Brunswick, R., Molina, D., & Bahro, M. (1996). Buspirone vs. haloperidol: A double-blind trial for agitation in a nursing home population with Alzheimer's disease. *American Journal of Geriatric Psychiatry, 4,* 263–267.

Clark, C.M., & Arnold, S.E. (1997). Alzheimer's disease. In R.E. Rakel (Ed.), *Conn's current therapy* (pp. 872–877). Philadelphia: W.B. Saunders.

Cummings, J.L., Gorman, D.G., & Shapira, J. (1993). Physostigmine ameliorates the delusions of Alzheimer's disease. *Biological Psychiatry, 33,* 536–541.

Fuchs, A., Hehnke, U., Erhart, C., Schell, C., Pramshohler, B., Danninger, B., & Schautzer, F. (1993). Video rating analysis of effect of maprotiline in patients with dementia and depression. *Pharmacopsychiatry, 26,* 37–41.

Gottlieb, G., McAllister, D., & Gur, R. (1988). Depot neuroleptics in the treatment of behavioral disorder in patients with Alzheimer's disease. *Journal of the American Geriatrics Society, 36,* 619–621.

Herrmann, N., & Eryavec, G. (1993). Buspirone in the management of agitation and aggression associated with dementia. *American Journal of Geriatric Psychiatry, 1*, 249–253.

Hyman, S.E., & Arana, G.W. (1987). *Handbook of psychiatric drug therapy* (pp. 115–123). Boston: Little, Brown.

Kanfer, D.I., Cummings, J.L., & Christine, D. (1996). Effect of tacrine on behavioral symptoms in Alzheimer's disease: An open-label study. *Journal of Geriatric Psychiatry and Neurology, 9*, 1–6.

Knapp, M.J., Knopman, D.S., Solomon, P.R., Pendelbury, W.W., Davis, C.S., & Gracon, S.I. (1994). A 30-week, randomized, controlled trial of high-dose tacrine in patients with Alzheimer's disease. *Journal of the American Medical Association, 271*, 985–991.

Knopman, D., Schneider, L., Davis, K., Talwalker, S., Smith, F., Hoover, T., & Gracon, S. (1996). Long-term tacrine (Cognex) treatment: Effects on nursing home placement and mortality. *Neurology, 47*, 166–177.

Kyomen, H.H., Nobel, K.W., & Wei, J.Y. (1991). The use of estrogen to decrease aggressive physical behavior in elderly men with dementia. *Journal of the American Geriatrics Society, 39*, 1110–1112.

LeBel, C.P., & Bondy, S.C. (1991). Oxygen radicals: Common mediators of neurotoxicity. *Neurotoxicology and Teratology, 13*, 341–346.

Lebert, F., Pasquier, F., & Petit, H. (1994). Behavioral effects of trazodone in Alzheimer's disease. *Journal of Clinical Psychiatry, 55*, 536–538.

Leibovici, A., & Tariot, P.N. (1988). Agitation associated with dementia: A systematic approach to treatment. *Psychopharmacology Bulletin, 24*, 49–53.

Lott, A.D., McElroy, S.L., & Keys, M.A. (1995). Valproate in the treatment of behavioral agitation in elderly patients with dementia. *Journal of Neuropsychiatry and Clinical Neuroscience, 7*, 314–319.

Madusoodanan, S., Brenner, R., Araujo, L., & Abaza, A. (1995). Efficacy of risperidone treatment for psychoses associated with schizophrenia, schizoaffective disorder, bipolar disorder, or senile dementia in 11 geriatric patients: A case series. *Journal of Clinical Psychiatry, 56*, 514–518.

National Institute on Aging. (1997). NIA Bulletin.

Nyth, A.L., & Gottfries, C.G. (1990). The clinical efficacy of citalopram in treatment of emotional disturbances in dementia disorders: A Nordic multi-center study. *British Journal of Psychiatry, 157*, 894–901.

Nyth, A.L., Gottfries, C.G., Lyby, K., Smedegaard-Andersen, L., Gylding-Sabroe, J., Kristensen, M., Refsom, H.E., Ofsti, E., Eriksson, S., & Syversen, S. (1992). A controlled, multi center, clinical study of citalopram and placebo in elderly, depressed patients with and without concomitant dementia. *Acta Psychiatrica Scandinavica, 86*, 138–145.

Reifler, B.V., Teri, L., Raskind, M., Veith, R., Barnes, R., White, E., & McLean, P. (1989). Double-blind trial of imipramine in Alzheimer's disease patients with and without depression. *American Journal of Psychiatry, 146*, 45–49.

Reisberg, B., Borenstein, J., Salob, S.B., Ferris, S.H., Franssen, E., & Georgotas, A. (1987). Behavioral symptoms in Alzheimer's disease: Phenomenology and treatment. *Journal of Clinical Psychiatry, 48*(Suppl. 5), 9–15.

Reyntgens, A., Heylen, S., Gelders, Y., Vanden Bussche, G., & Janssen, P.A. (1988). Risperidone in the treatment of behavioral symptoms in psychogeriatric patients: A pilot clinical investigation. *Psychopharmacology, 96*, 335.

Rogers, F.L., Friedhoff, L.T., & the Donepezil Study Group. (1996). The efficacy and safety of donepezil in patients with Alzheimer's disease: Results of a U.S. multicenter randomized, double-blind, placebo-controlled trial. *Dementia, 7*, 293–303.

Rogers, J., Kirby, L.C., Hempelman, S.R., Berry, D.L., McGeer, P.L., Kaszniak, A.W., Zalinski, J., Cofield, M., Mansukhani, L., Willson, P., & Kogan, F. (1993). Clinical trial of indomethacin in Alzheimer's disease. *Neurology, 43*, 1609–1611.

Salzman, C., Vaccaro, B., Leiff, J., & Weiner, A. (1995). Clozapine in older patients with psychosis and behavioral disruption. *Geriatric Psychiatry, 3*, 26–33.

Sano, M., Ernesto, C., Thomas, R.G., Klauber, M.R., Schafer, K., Grundman, M., et al. (in press). A two-year, double-blind, randomized, multicenter trial of selegiline and alpha-tocopherol in the treatment of Alzheimer's disease. *New England Journal of Medicine.*

Satlin, A. (1994). Sleep disorders in dementia. *Psychiatry Annual, 24*, 186–190.

Schneider, L.S. (1996). New therapeutic approaches to Alzheimer's disease. *Journal of Clinical Psychiatry, 57*(Suppl. 14), 30–36.

Schneider, L.S., & Olin, J.T. (1994). Overview of clinical trials of hydergine in dementia. *Archives of Neurology, 51*, 787–798.

Schneider, L.S., Pollock, V.E., & Lyness, S.A. (1990). A meta analysis of controlled trials of neuroleptic treatment in dementia. *Journal of the American Geriatrics Society, 38*, 553–563.

Schneider, L.S., & Tariot, P.N. (1994). Emerging drugs for Alzheimer's disease: Mechanisms of action and prospects for cognitive enhancing medications. *Medical Clinics of North America, 78*, 911–934.

Shaw, S.H., Curson, H., & Coquetin, J.P. (1992). A double-blind comparative study of Zolpidem and placebo in the treatment of insomnia in elderly psychiatric in-patients. *Journal of Internal Medicine Research, 20*, 150–161.

Sherwin, B.B. (1994). Estrogenic effects on memory in women. *Annals of the New York Academy of Science, 743*, 213–230.

Singer, C., McArthur, A., Hughes, R., Sack, R., Kaye, J., & Lewy, A. (1995). High dose melatonin administration and sleep in the elderly. *Sleep Research, 24A*, 151.

Sival, R.C., Haffmens, P.M.J., Van Gent, P.P., & van Nieuwker, J.F. (1994). The effects of sodium valproate on disturbed behavior in dementia. *Journal of the American Geriatrics Society, 42*, 906–907.

Stewart, W.F., Kawas, C., Corrada, M., & Metter, E.J. (1997). Risk of Alzheimer's disease and duration of NSAID use. *Neurology, 48*, 626–632.

Sultzer, D.L., Gray, K.F., Gunay, I., Berisford, M.A., & Mahler, M.E. (1997). A double-blind comparison of trazodone and haloperidol for treatment of agitation in patients with dementia. *American Journal of Geriatric Psychiatry, 5*, 60–69.

Sunderland, P., Molchan, F., Lawlor, B., Martinez, R., Mellow, A., Martinson, H., Putman, K., & Lalonde, F. (1992). A strategy of "combination chemotherapy" in Alzheimer's disease: Rational and preliminary results with physostigmine plus deprenyl. *International Psychogeriatrics, 4*(Suppl. 2), 291–309.

Tariot, P.N., Cohen, R.M., Sunderland, T., Newhouse, P.A., Young, D., Mellow, A.M., et al. (1987). L-Deprenyl in Alzheimer's disease: Preliminary evidence for behavioral change with monoamine oxidase-B inhibition. *Archives of General Psychiatry, 44*, 427–433.

Tariot, P.N., Erb, R., Leibovic, A., Podgorski, C.A., Cox, C., Asnis, J., Kolassa, J., & Irvine, C. (1994). Carbamazepine treatment of agitation in nursing home patients with dementia: A preliminary study. *Journal of the American Geriatrics Society, 42*, 1160–1166.

Tune, L.E., Steel, C., & Cooper, T. (1991). Neuroleptic drugs in the management of behavioral symptoms of Alzheimer's disease. *Psychiatric Clinics of North America, 14*, 353–373.

IV

Special Management Challenges

13

Eating—Mealtime Challenges and Interventions

Carly R. Hellen, OTR/L

Mealtime and the eating process can challenge the abilities and reflect the disabilities of older adults with dementia. Residents who exhibit difficult behaviors at meals rarely try to create problems. Their conduct is often a manifestation of their communication system: The residents' personality, reactions to stressful situations, and dementia itself combine to produce unwanted responses. The dining room becomes an arena in which behaviors are revealed, responses need to be facilitated and supported, and demeanor is exhibited that calls for problem solving and refocusing. Mealtime, therefore, is more than simply a time to meet nutritional needs; it is of primary importance when caring for residents with Alzheimer's disease. Mealtime represents a communion of cherished memories of special people, celebrations, and events joined with the sharing of food. Carrying on these traditions and rituals, the giving and receiving of food, and good nutrition, along with engendering feelings of security and support in the nursing facility, can promote a sense of connectedness or wellness in residents with Alzheimer's disease.

EMPOWERING RESIDENTS TO EAT

Eating capabilities vary in response to health status and changes that occur as the dementia progresses, to caregivers, and to the environment. Focusing on what residents can do rather than what they cannot do demands that staff enter the residents' world. Thus, the paradigm shifts from the typical medical model of *doing for* or *doing to* the residents and becomes a humanistic model of *doing with* the residents. Staff may need to introduce specific interventions to ensure that residents successfully consume a meal.

UTILIZE RESIDENTS' EATING HISTORY AND LIFESTORY

Assessment of residents' eating capabilities begins with knowledge of their premorbid eating history and life story, which can be compiled in a LifeStory Book (see Appendix). If residents are unable to provide information, their family or caregiver may be able to offer insights. Learning residents' eating preferences is crucial because foods and mealtime memories provide a link to the present. Often, disliked foods and consistencies continue to be rejected. The LifeStory Book may benefit caregivers as a behavioral refocusing intervention, especially the information contained within that is related to favorite traditions, family roles, and cultural influences that surround mealtimes.

IDENTIFY BEHAVIORAL CHALLENGES TO EATING

Difficult behaviors at mealtime evolve from residents' cognitive, physical, psychosocial, and environmental responses. Using problem-solving tools such as the Sensory Profile, the Behavior Profile, and the Behavior Tracking Form (see Appendix) can assist caregivers in identifying the specific difficult behavior and its possible cause.

FACILITATE ABILITIES TO REDUCE EATING DIFFICULTIES

Continual assessment of residents' changing capabilities and limitations is paramount in order to refocus adverse eating behaviors and to weave their strengths into a plan of action. By simplifying and modifying foods and dining apparatus, residents may experience success and feel valued. Difficult behaviors can be reduced when residents feel safe and find their abilities appreciated. Implementation of supportive care may be necessary when residents cannot initiate self-monitoring of needs.

DECREASE ANTECEDENTS TO DIFFICULT BEHAVIORS

Undesirable behaviors that perpetuate residents' disabilities often can be avoided if their particular antecedent is prevented or reduced. To that end, changes in the actual mealtime, foods, and environment may be necessary. Thus, prevention is the key to a positive mealtime experience.

EMPOWER STAFF WHO EXEMPLIFY SENSITIVITY

Caregivers must demonstrate patience and sensitivity. Staff who are respected, encouraged to solve problems, and given the necessary managerial support are empowered to move into the residents' world of ability and need. Hurried, harassed, and unappreciated staff often find enabling residents' abilities impossible when their own strengths and abilities are disregarded.

Ensuring adequate nutritional intake for people with dementia requires creative approaches and interventions by staff such as the following:

1. Multisensory cueing—Combining cues from all five senses helps to orient residents to the task of eating and helps them to be more attentive to it (e.g., the caregiver inserts a small spoonful of mashed potatoes into a resident's mouth, then places the spoon in the person's hand and gives simple instructions to place the spoon into the potatoes and bring the spoon up to the mouth—employing gustatory, visual, auditory, and tactile senses).

2. Task simplification and sequencing—Simplification of a task by breaking it up into multiple steps to be performed one at a time in a functional order may facilitate residents' involvement.

3. Mirroring—Copying what someone else is doing can guide people with dementia to participate actively by reflecting what they have observed. For example, a caregiver raising a spoonful of soup to her own mouth may be imitated. The objectives of mirroring are to obtain residents' attention, use words and motions to copy the activity, and encourage them to do the same for themselves.

4. Hand-over-hand approach—A caregiver places his or her hand over the hand of a resident and steers it from the food to the mouth and then back to the food. This technique helps residents feel a sense of accomplishment, as though they were self-feeding.

5. Chaining and end-chaining—Chaining occurs when residents are able to take over after the caregiver initiates the activity using the hand-over-hand approach. At times, chaining may need to be reapplied if residents stop self-feeding. End-chaining provides a cue at the completion of the intended task to influence residents to continue independently. For example, Jannise puts the spoonful of mashed potatoes into John's mouth and then lets go of the spoon, allowing it to remain in his mouth. When John becomes aware or annoyed enough that he has a strange object sticking out of his mouth, he raises his hand to the spoon. Jannise's action may be what is needed to reconnect John to the task of eating so that he is able to continue self-feeding. If he stops eating, the end-chaining can be repeated.

6. Bridging—Bridging is a method of sensory connection. A resident holds the same object while a caregiver carries out the task. The purpose is to provide focus, increase attention span, and reduce anxiety. When bridging occurs,

residents become better centered on the eating activity and, therefore, more cooperative.

7. Eating facilitation techniques—Staff can use the following techniques:

- Mouth-opening assistance: Place fingers under resident's jaw; using a firm motion, press up quickly; release fingers
- Lip-opening assistance: Gently but firmly use thumb and fingers to squeeze lips together; release fingers
- Swallowing assistance: Gently stroke resident's throat in an upward motion from the base of the neck toward the jaw
- Increasing oral stimulation: Use ice
- Food bolus: Use correct-size food bolus (i.e., amount of food in a bite)

ABILITY-BASED NUTRITIONAL CARE

The changes that occur during the progression of Alzheimer's disease affect people cognitively, physically, and emotionally and spiritually, and present environmental challenges as well. Continual monitoring and assessment by the caregiver is required to identify these changes in order to modify or prevent difficult behavior. Residents' positive responses must be promoted in an environment that adapts to their constantly changing abilities.

COGNITIVE CHALLENGES AND POSSIBILITIES

Dementia includes approximately 70 progressive, irreversible diseases that cause losses of cognition, orientation to time and space, alterations in emotion, and ability to perform voluntary activities. Each disease causes different behavioral symptoms depending on the area of the brain affected, the location and size of damage, the premorbid personality, the person's culture/ethnicity, and environmental stressors (Hall, 1994).

Dementia leads the person through several stages, each with its own characteristics and challenges to the eating process. From the stages of forgetfulness and confusion to the end-stage of impending death, provisions must be made by caregivers to encourage adequate nutrition for people with dementia. Provision of community services and home health aides may be considered in the early stages of the dementing disease, even when the person still seems independent and able to prepare meals at home. These older adults may be anxious about meal planning and shopping and may prepare the same foods repeatedly in order to eliminate the need for making choices. Safety factors also should be taken into consideration when people with dementia cook in their own home. Confusion could cause inappropriate items to be heated and forgetfulness could lead to a fire hazard (Hall, 1994).

Residents' level of orientation and awareness combine with their remaining cognitive abilities to create success or difficulties during the eating process. Misbehavior evolves from the frustration of feeling disconnected from expectations—their own and the caregiver's. Because of the continual regression in retention of what was previously learned, verbal and behavioral cues must be offered in order for the person's attention to remain on the meal (Warden et al., 1995).

Table 1 presents five common cognitive challenges to mealtime success and interventions that can be used to ensure success.

PHYSICAL CHALLENGES AND POSSIBILITIES

Physical challenges related to medical disabilities are apraxia, dysphagia, and excess disabilities. Apraxia, the inability to plan or carry out meaningful movement, may limit residents' ability to self-feed. Dysphagia may hinder a person's ability to swallow (Kayser-Jones & Schell, 1997). Excess disabilities occur when problems, situations (e.g., physical or psychological difficulties, overstimulation from the environment), or illness affect residents by escalating dementia-related difficulties. Other possible causes of excess disabilities such as fatigue, anemia, dehydration, undiagnosed fractures, urinary or bowel retention, and seizures may precipitate behaviors that affect nutrition.

Pacing, wandering, and being restless interfere with eating at mealtimes and can lead to unwanted side effects. People with dementia often reflect their wellness and behavioral adjustment with loss or gain of weight. Some weight loss in people with dementia occurs when they pace excessively for extended periods of time; increased nutritional support is required. As many as 1,600 extra calories can be needed above the Recommended Dietary Allowance to maintain the current weight of residents who pace. Caregiver attempts to keep residents seated can cause combativeness and increase residents' anxiety.

Table 2 presents four common physical challenges to mealtime success and interventions that can be used to ensure success.

PSYCHOSOCIAL AND EMOTIONAL CHALLENGES AND POSSIBILITIES

Difficult behaviors exhibited by residents during mealtime may arise from their feelings of fear and loss. Residents' families, staff, and the facility's dietary department and administration must work together to provide a calm environment for mealtime, foods and utensils that residents can use successfully, and well-trained staff who know the residents' strengths and their difficulties. Table 3 presents six common psychosocial and emotional challenges to mealtime success and interventions that can be used to ensure success.

ENVIRONMENTAL CHALLENGES AND POSSIBILITIES

Environmental competency requires ongoing assessment, flexibility, and creativity. Table 4 presents three common environmental challenges to mealtime success and interventions that can be used to ensure success.

TABLE 1.   COGNITIVE CHALLENGES TO MEALTIME SUCCESS AND SUCCESSFUL INTERVENTIONS

FORGETFULNESS AND DISORIENTATION

Challenge	Intervention
Misinterprets the bodily needs of hunger and thirst	Offer water and liquids constantly. Residents usually do not ask for a drink, and dehydration may increase combativeness.
Plays with food Forgets how to eat Does not recognize food as food	At times, residents cannot move on from the before-meal activity to the meal itself. Consequently, they play with food because there are no cueing devices to inform them of the change. As an intervention, alter the appearance of the table to signal that the activity is now eating by using a tablecloth, flowers, baskets for napkins, and place mats.
	Provide a multisensory approach: for example, use aromas such as coffee, cinnamon toast, or bacon to cue for breakfast; soups (especially onion) and baking bread for lunch; pasta sauce, cake, or pie for dinner. Beckoning with an item of food may prompt a reluctant resident to the dining area.
Eats with fingers instead of utensils	Increase the number of finger foods being offered (see Appendix). Positively affirm residents' eating abilities. Simplify the eating task so they can succeed, using one-step directions as needed.
Does not use utensils correctly (Kayser-Jones & Schell, 1997)	Limit the number of utensils. Often, residents with dementia eat with a knife because they pick it up with their dominant hand to cut their food (whether or not it needs to be cut) and then forget to put it down to select a fork or a spoon.
Unable to make choices if too much food or too many containers are present at one time	Serve one course at a time so the necessity of making choices is limited and there are fewer distractions available. When appropriate, allow menu selection and choice between 2–3 main courses. If dining at a restaurant, offer the menu and give the cueing needed to help with choices. For example, "Would you prefer chicken or beef today?" If residents cannot make choices at all and you know their likes and dislikes, you might say, "This restaurant is noted for their excellent roast beef. Would you like some?"

Demonstrates an inability to understand what is expected of them at mealtime

If residents feel that there is too much food on their plate, use two plates, serving half a meal at a time.

LIMITED ATTENTION SPAN

Challenge

Inability to attend to the task of eating limits the meal being consumed entirely

Intervention

Use simple words. Touch and redirect the resident to the task of eating.

Starts and stops the eating process off and on throughout the meal

Leaves the table during the meal

Five to six meals may be needed for residents who are unable to eat much at any one time because they become agitated when caregivers try to refocus them.

The meal may be a combination of sitting and eating, followed by walking and eating finger foods from a bowl. Make sandwiches of anything that will hold together (mashed potatoes make good glue). Waist pouches may help a pacer to keep his hands free so he can hold finger foods (Hall, 1994).

Falls asleep while eating

Bridging encourages residents to focus and increase limited attention span. Having them hold a spoon or plastic cup during the feeding process helps when they are total feeders.

Takes mood-controlling medications

Psychoactive drugs may intensify chewing and swallowing difficulties, or simply make residents too sleepy to eat (Hall, 1994).

JUDGMENT AND SAFETY

Challenge

Eats food pieces that are too big to swallow safely

Intervention

Assess food pieces for size, thickness, and consistency; make necessary adjustments.

(continued)

199

TABLE 1—*continued*

JUDGMENT AND SAFETY—*continued*

Challenge

Overstuffs the mouth

Eats nonedibles or spoiled food

Pours liquids onto foods

Drinks or eats scalding liquids or food

Takes another resident's food

Bites down too hard on utensils

Intervention

If food stuffing occurs, and the mouth is already full, work with OT/ST to assess and develop a plan.

Avoid garnishes that are not easily chewed or eaten, or that are merely decorative and inedible. If needed, put in place a written policy and procedure to support this safety measure.

If residents constantly pour liquids over the food, it may be necessary to provide them only when food is not present.

Serve food only at a temperature warm enough to avoid burning the mouth.

Offer visual cueing for boundaries by using place mats to reduce interest in another's meal. Square tables provide better definition of territory than round tables.

Avoid plastic utensils; biting down on them can cause splintering. If biting down occurs, speak softly to the resident, and gently stroke large extensor muscles (e.g., the back of the arm). Do not pull on the utensil; try the mouth-opening facilitation intervention or offer a drink. Use metal spoons covered with smooth latex or rubber to limit damage to teeth.

PERCEPTUAL DYSFUNCTION

Challenge

Shows signs of agnosia (i.e., not understanding or misinterpreting information coming in from the senses; therefore, the cognitive awareness is not being integrated, and the reaction is compromised)

Intervention

Use the Sensory Profile (see Appendix) to identify needs and ways to supply redundant cues for all of the senses. For example, the resident may not realize that the soup is food. Use the word *soup*; bring it up for them to smell; lift a spoonful up, and then let it splash back into the bowl; offer a small spoonful to the lips to get a taste and feel its warmth.

Avoid inedibles that may look like food. For example, a white napkin may look like a slice of bread; vanilla ice cream or milk in a Styrofoam cup may not be seen or may lead to the cup being eaten also.

Shows figure-ground discrimination dysfunction

Focus on color contrast in terms of the food to the plate or cup and the contrast of the plate to the place mat. Supporting visual interpretation can reduce residents' anxiety.

COMMUNICATION: UNDERSTANDING AND BEING UNDERSTOOD

Interventions

Use the resident's LifeStory book and listing of food preferences and dislikes as cueing devices when residents do not understand the caregiver's directions or what is expected of them.

Use multisensory cueing with frequent pointing. Lift the item away from the table or food up from the plate to regain recognition.

Use verbal encouragement: "I cooked this chicken just for you," or "This is a new recipe I want to cook for my husband. Would you please try it for me and tell me what you think?"

When asking questions about food choices, use "either/or" questions rather than questions requiring yes/no responses, which could lead to "no's" and not eating. Do not count on the residents' verbalizations; constantly observe and monitor the eating process, making any necessary adjustments.

Try to provide consistency in caregiving. A Swedish study reports that in the course of 1 month, up to 30 different caregivers were observed helping a single resident at mealtime (Kayser-Jones & Schell, 1997).

TABLE 2. PHYSICAL CHALLENGES TO MEALTIME SUCCESS AND SUCCESSFUL INTERVENTIONS

EXCESS DISABILITIES

Challenge	Intervention
Sensory-deficit needs not met	Assess and reduce excess disability factors affecting residents' unwanted behaviors. Sensory deficits can be assessed by using the Sensory Profile (see Appendix) to determine residents' abilities and disabilities involving vision, hearing, smell, taste, and response to touch. If prosthetic devices are used, they must be in good working order and specific to the problem. For example, just because a resident has glasses on, do not assume that sight is completely adjusted, that the glasses are clean, or that the right glasses are on the right resident. If hearing aids are not tolerated, ask residents to wear only one so that the sound input is easier for them to integrate into meaningfulness. Check dentures for proper fit and make necessary adjustments and referrals. If these devices are not well tolerated, assess the situation to see whether wearing them only at mealtimes works.
Chronic pain or discomfort	Staff should work with residents' physicians to use scheduled medications (rather than PRNs) for chronic pain intervention. Many residents cannot correctly identify or report pain. When arthritic pain involves the finger joints or the grasp is affected, a foam tube from a hair curler can be slipped onto the utensil to increase the grasp ability and promote proprioception (i.e., awareness of the object being held).
Onset of an illness	Check residents' clothing, incontinent product, and general health factors prior to the meal. Irritation stemming from discomfort or the onset of an infection interferes with eating. During flu season or at times when several residents have infections, take temperatures daily using an ear thermometer—intervene before residents act out their illnesses by refusing to eat or by demonstrating a change in their eating pattern.
Presence of chronic disability due to arthritis, CVA, Parkinson's disease or similar symptoms, or fatigue	Parkinson's disease or Parkinsonian symptoms can produce problems in swallowing and balance, and hand tremor. Arm rigidity can affect the spoon's movement from food to mouth. Frustration, leading to acting-out behaviors, often can be refocused if heavy or weighted utensils are used to reduce tremors. Cups or mugs for soups or liquids,

scoop bowls, a grip mat, or a damp cloth under the plate prevent sliding and can decrease residents' anxiety. Hand-over-hand assistance or either form of chaining may help to initiate the movement of utensil to mouth. Adding unsalted broths can facilitate swallowing.

Residents may be assessed as demonstrating stubborn or difficult behaviors when the response is actually related to Parkinson's disease, which can exhibit an off/on cycle. This cycle is related to the timing of medications and the residents' response to them. For example, residents may be able to eat lunch independently but cannot carry out the activity of eating dinner.

Residents with stroke and dementia can become agitated during the eating process for several reasons. By using the resident's clock drawings,[1] you can assess their perceptual distortions and position the food for visual needs and easy access. Finger foods (see Appendix) should be used if residents are forced to eat with their nondominant hand and are having difficulty. Work with the OT/PT/ST to determine needed assistance with positioning, food consistency, and appropriately adapted equipment. However, try to avoid adapted equipment if possible because, often, it becomes an object or focus of interest, distracting residents from eating.

MECHANICS OF EATING

Challenge

Utensil to the food and the mouth

Difficulty opening mouth

Difficulty closing mouth

Stuffs mouth without swallowing; pouching

Intervention

Practice mirroring, chaining, and bridging.

Facilitation can open the mouth, or ask the resident to say, "Ahhhh." Sometimes yawning in their face causes them to yawn and opens their mouth.

Some residents may chew a piece of meat and then spit it out. Softer meat or purée may need to be used.

Implement a soft-food or a puréed diet. Massage residents' jaw.

(continued)

203

TABLE 2—*continued*

MECHANICS OF EATING—*continued*

Challenge

Eats too fast
Does not chew
Chews one bite for a long time
Has swallowing dysfunction
Chokes

Has periodontal disease; oral discomfort

Intervention

Choking problems must be assessed by a speech-language pathologist. However, usually a tableside evaluation is sufficient. Residents with advanced dementia have limited ability to follow through in a cookie-swallow test. All staff must be trained in the Heimlich maneuver. At times, sounding like a stern taskmaster may help; for example, "Henry, swallow right now," said with insistence.

Practice routine dental care and oral hygiene. Residents may not tolerate dentures but can still gum their food.

CONTINUOUS, UNPRODUCTIVE MOVEMENT AND NOISE

Challenge

Paces and refuses to sit down
Leaves the table throughout the meal
Stands up and sits down

Bangs on tables
Flails arms
Yells or screams during mealtime

Intervention

A geri-chair with a lapboard or other type of restraint chair may offer a solution if residents can tolerate it. (Certainly a physician's order is mandated, and the residents must be released as soon as the meal ends.) Residents may like the feeling of being secure, of not having to initiate their own sense of boundaries, or of perceiving the cueing that they do not need to get up and serve the food.

Banging, yelling, flailing arms, or screaming can be signs of distress or attempts at self-stimulation. Using a Walkman with quiet music and large earpieces may help.

WEIGHT GAIN/LOSS

Intervention

Residents who exceed their recommended body weight without ambulation problems have a weight reserve. Weight reserve may make the difference between recovery and continued disability if a fall, broken bone, or illness affects the residents' ability to eat. Weighing residents weekly or at least twice a month helps staff to assess needs; weight cannot be measured accurately by monthly monitoring.

Doubling up on breakfast may help weight to be maintained.

Weight loss may call for between-meal snacks. Offering snacks mid-morning, mid-afternoon, and before bedtime is suggested.

Although a tray may contain little food after mealtime, it does not mean that most of the food was eaten. Note whether food may have been wasted through spillage by residents (Kayser-Jones & Schell, 1997).

A CAT (consistency as tolerated) order allows staff to assess residents for appropriate food consistency. At times, a meal with two types of food consistencies may need to be used during one mealtime, with residents moving back and forth between the foods. Foods that have a smooth consistency may be more acceptable.

Alternating hot and cold foods helps to trigger swallowing.

Establish a policy and procedure so that honey or sugar may be used on food, if medically appropriate; these condiments may help to entice residents to eat. Because people with end-stage Alzheimer's disease usually favor sweets, they can be enticed to eat by adding sweet thickeners to their foods.

High-protein and increased-calorie foods are useful. Check liquid supplements with the dietitian for the protein content because some products are held in the stomach for a lengthy period of time. For example, John does not eat well at breakfast, so he receives a liquid supplement around 10:00 A.M. If the substance is still in his stomach when lunch arrives, John will not eat well at lunch, which will start John on a habit of not eating solid food. Continue with regular food for as long as possible. Recipes for nutrient-dense foods are available (see Appendix).

---

[1]By asking the resident to draw a clock face on a plain piece of paper, the caregiver can use the spacing of the numbers to assess the resident's perceptual abilities or difficulties. For example, if all of the numbers are on one side of the clock, the resident's food should be served toward that side. A similar assessment is to observe the resident during mealtime: Does he or she eat only from one side of the plate? If the plate is rotated, does the resident then eat the remaining portion?

TABLE 3. PSYCHOSOCIAL/EMOTIONAL CHALLENGES TO MEALTIME SUCCESS AND SUCCESSFUL INTERVENTIONS

FEARFULNESS

Challenge	Intervention
Fear of not being fed	Provide assurance to residents that they are safe and that you are "there" for them. If they cannot tolerate being served last, make adjustments.
Fear of food being poisoned	Serve food in a Styrofoam take-out container or a sealed container. Tell residents that the food has been ordered especially for them. Avoid mixing any kind of medication into the food because this may increase their concern about being poisoned. Sometimes simply changing their eating area helps relieve their worries. Avoid arguing or trying to explain the situation at length. Suspiciousness can also arise if residents see that their meal is different from that of their table mates. Having food look the same can help reduce concern; puréed foods can be sculpted in molds to look like the "real" thing. Fearfulness can also occur if dessert is given at an inappropriate point during the meal.

ANXIETY

Challenge	Intervention
Someone seated in "their place"	Some residents prefer or demand to have exactly the same seat for each meal and will become aggressive if someone is in their seat. Place cards can be used, or residents' chairs can be removed until just before they arrive at the table.
Sits too close to others or someone they dislike; dislike of the person assisting them	Be aware of residents' preferred table mates. If someone is disliked or causes discomfort, eating will be affected. Staff should also be alert to making a last-minute seating change if an unhappy incident occurs just before the meal between two residents who normally enjoy each other's company. Staff may need to sit between residents who openly dislike each other or when there is unrest at a table. An acceptable peer group for eating is important. Sitting too close to another person can cause aggravation.

Being rushed to the table; not having enough time to finish the meal

Must wait too long to eat

Avoid having the food arrive early. Prevent aggravation by allotting enough time for meals.

Avoid waiting at the table for a period of time without food being served. Some residents behave better if they are not taken into the dining area until the meal is completely set up. Singing or word games may help decrease waiting intolerance.

Agitation

Eliminate caffeine.

DEPRESSED AFFECT AND APATHY

Challenge

A depressed mood may limit eating responses, perhaps causing food to sit in the mouth without being swallowed; there may be limited physical movement and a decreased interest in food

Intervention

Hand-over-hand feeding may help connect residents to the activity. A pleasant seating area, including light, sound, attractiveness of the food, and friends seated at the table, may help to stimulate eating.

CONCERNS AND PRIDE

Challenge

No money to pay for meal

Intervention

Issue meal tickets, "credit cards," or have a bill filled out with a receipt to help residents with "no money" to accept the meal. Photocopy money in color for residents to use, or tell them that the meal is paid for by insurance. Inform them that the meal is part of the club membership; therefore, it is required that they eat dinner at the club on a daily basis.

(continued)

TABLE 3—*continued*

CONCERNS AND PRIDE—*continued*

Challenge	Intervention
Hospitality needs unmet; people present but not eating	Everybody, including family members, staff, any visitors, and even surveyors in the area, should be seated during the meal unless they are involved in passing food or assisting someone. A policy of safeguarding residents from stressful situations can be written to provide the rationale behind the insistence that everyone be seated. Residents often express concern if people at their table are not eating. Therefore, anyone seated and assisting at a table should have a cup of juice or coffee and perhaps some toast or crackers, so it looks like he or she is being included in the meal. At times, the best way to help residents to eat is for staff to join them and eat the same meal.
Feeling they are volunteers and do not deserve to eat	If residents feel that they cannot eat because they are volunteers at the facility, assure them that they have worked hard and deserve a meal.
Feeling too much is being done for them	Residents' pride is diminished when food is cut up or items on the tray are prepared to be eaten in front of them. They feel that they are "nonpeople" or that they have no abilities. Preparing the food in an area removed from residents helps them to uphold their self-esteem.

FAMILY RELATIONSHIPS

Challenge	Intervention
Dislikes person present	The mere presence of certain family members may cause residents to become anxious and not eat. If this becomes an ongoing situation, the relative must be asked not to be present at mealtime.
Family too insistent on or does not encourage eating	Monitoring family members helps to reduce agitation. Some family members feed residents too fast or too slow, are insistent that they eat everything, or are not insistent enough.

Family interferes with appropriate diet

Problems can occur if family members bring along foods residents should not have, supply foods high in sugar (especially before meals), or eat from residents' plates—tell them not to bring such foods and explain to them why they should not eat off the residents' plates.

PROBLEMATIC MIND-SET

Challenge	Intervention
"Mother–Martyr" mind-set (everyone must be served first; will go without food if food is limited)	Assure residents that there is plenty of food. Keep their foods warm while others are being served. Residents with this mind-set should eat first when possible. At other times, they may need to eat long after the other residents or in another location, such as standing in the serving area.
"I'm too fat"	People with dementia often remember past struggles with weight and endless dieting. Tell them that you serve only low-fat, low-calorie diet food that has been selected especially for them by their doctor. A table for "weight watchers" can be set up but all must be served the same "diet" foods.
"Depression-era" mentality (will eat only part of the meal and save the rest for later; puts food in pockets, purse)	Monitor the residents' clothing and room for stored food.
Decision to "give up"	Some residents appear to have the ability to choose to stop eating and will do so. "Eating out," even in another area of the facility, may reignite interest in eating. Setting up a "breakfast club" with personal invitations also often works. Taking the food away and then returning it a few moments later may help if they have forgotten that they had already been offered food. Spouses should always be encouraged to order a tray of food to share with their loved one. Assess all variables—foods, other residents, staff, family, noise, and the environment (see "Nutritional Challenges in Late-Stage Care").

TABLE 4. ENVIRONMENTAL CHALLENGES TO MEALTIME SUCCESS AND SUCCESSFUL INTERVENTIONS

UNDERSTIMULATION

Challenge	Intervention
Overly quiet environment; bland food	At times, complete quiet or a sterile environment can increase agitation, causing residents to wonder if they are in the right place at the right time, doing the right thing. Residents with dementia usually appreciate a friendly environment (including the dining area and all of its components) that is pleasant and comfortable.

OVERSTIMULATION

Challenge	Intervention
Too much noise, color, or movement; alarm or intercom noise; irritating resident, staff, and/or family; movement (no matter the source, noise can cause problem behavior and lessen the possibility of a successful mealtime experience)	Sit quietly, close your eyes, and listen to the activity at mealtime to assess the noise level. Locate the offending sounds and make the necessary changes. Determine at each mealtime whether soft music is a positive or negative stimulus.
Furniture is too close and confining	The actual dining area will irritate residents if it is cramped and limits movement. Dining areas that have an alcove for quieter and less-stimulating dining are helpful.
Television is on	Often, residents with dementia have a "black and white" interpretation of what they see and hear. For example, the house they see burning on television is their house, or the child who is crying is their child. Overheard conversation among staff, family, and other residents can be interpreted similarly. Residents may become too distracted and overstimulated to eat, or they get up and want to tend to the perceived problem. Monitor background noise.

Dining Area, Equipment

Challenge

Room size and setup; type and sizes of tables; chairs, lighting, window glare, dishes, glassware, and utensils cause disruptive behavior

Intervention

Having a variety of tables is an excellent way to adapt to needs. For example, a table for two or for one may be needed if a resident is expressing hostility or paranoia. The same is true with the placement of tables in the environment: Square tables can be pushed together for different groupings of residents. Often, round tables increase the incidents of residents' eating from another person's plate. Some residents cannot tolerate or eat successfully in a crowded area and may feel better with an over-the-bed–type table that is located away from others.

Glare from windows and window reflections, especially at night, can cause agitation. Be careful that seating never faces windows because the pupils of older eyes have difficulty adjusting to the visual field of the food on the table from the glare.

Scents can have a positive effect on residents' abilities, facilitating them, or they may have a negative effect, leading to acting out behaviors. Well-accepted scents to try are baking bread, cinnamon and cloves, or freshly popped corn.

To limit frustration, provide cups and glassware that are easy to grasp. Good options are cups with straws or sippy cups and utensils of varying sizes and weights. Rubber-coated baby spoons may be less offensive to residents than large spoons when placed in the mouth and provide a protective shield for residents who bite down on utensils. An adequate supply of these spoons, napkins, and food thickeners should be accessible when feeding a resident. A deep-dish plate can be beneficial because residents can push the utensil against the edge while trying to load food onto a fork or spoon.

NUTRITIONAL CHALLENGES IN LATE-STAGE DEMENTIA CARE

In the final phases of Alzheimer's disease, many residents develop eating problems because of damage to the brain cells that regulate eating and swallowing functions (Warden et al., 1995). Often, residents lose weight and become malnourished. Vitamin, mineral, and protein deficiencies increase residents' susceptibility to systemic infections and other health problems.

A person with late-stage dementia may refuse to eat for numerous reasons, including the exhibition of behaviors that interfere with successful eating such as biting down on utensils, holding food in the mouth, spitting food out, or pushing the caregiver's hand or food-filled utensil away. Even in the terminal stage, residents' behaviors can be a demonstration of control, permitting or not allowing food to enter their mouth. Some residents simply may not remember how to eat (Warden et al., 1995).

Choking, on both food and liquid, creates a special category of feeding difficulties and critical concerns. When aspiration pneumonia is likely, a frequent inclination is to place the person on a feeding tube. However, this practice can be misleading. Research shows that nasogastric tube feeding may increase aspiration pneumonia because of an increased risk of reflux of stomach contents into the esophagus (Warden et al., 1995). In many situations tube feeding may be substituted with proper natural feeding techniques. Oral feeding adds to individuals' quality of life and allows them to enjoy the flavor of food. In addition, the discomfort caused by the tube and the possible necessity of restraints should be considered: In one case at the Edith Nourse Rogers Memorial Veterans' Hospital in Bedford, Massachusetts, an individual with Alzheimer's disease, who was completely disoriented and speech impaired, improved dramatically when his feeding tube was replaced with natural feeding under close monitoring by his caregiver. After repetitive cueing techniques, the man improved remarkably, both verbally and physically (Warden et al., 1995).

Interventions must be individualized to meet the unique requirements of each resident. Caregivers must focus attention on residents and face them using cogent eye contact. Residents should be maintained in a position appropriate to prevent choking—upright, with the head centered and forward over the midline of the body (Warden et al., 1995). In the later stages of dementia, the sucking reflex may become more apparent; toddlers' cups with spouted lids or straws may be useful in aiding swallowing (Hall, 1994). Many times, weight is lost, even when all of the allotted food is consumed. The quality of the nutrition becomes paramount. Caregivers should aim to provide the highest nutrient intake with the lowest volume of food. Appropriate hydration is mandatory.

Families should be working with social services well before residents' need for late-stage dementia care. At this time, difficult behaviors become more of a physiologically induced response than a demonstration of reactions to self and activities of daily living. End-of-life decisions include planning for the delivery of nutritional needs and hydration. Hospice services can be employed. During the final days and hours of residents' lives, caring, support, and respect can provide an empathic connection among residents, families, and staff.

CONCLUSION

The wellness of and nutritional support for people with dementia require difficult behaviors to be refocused. Creativity and flexibility are the hallmarks of a successful eating program, and these qualities need to be applied to all aspects of both the foods being served and the activity at mealtime. Dedicated caregivers who are sensitive, patient, and willing to adapt are committed to facilitating a good quality of life for people with dementia. They will support residents' abilities and help to reduce difficult behaviors. Caregivers will feel gifted with the awareness that they have extended a caring hand and spirit to their residents.

REFERENCES

Hall, G.R. (1994, April). Chronic dementia: Challenges in feeding a patient. *Journal of Gerontological Nursing, 20,* 21–30.

Kayser-Jones, J., & Schell, E. (1997, July). The mealtime experience of a cognitively impaired elder: Ineffective and effective strategies. *Journal of Gerontological Nursing,* 23(7), 33–39.

Warden, V., Glennon, M., Morrison, J., Payne, M., Smith, S., Whittaker, J., Brennan, R., Fiorintine, A., Papile, L., Hurley, A., Volicer, L., & Archambault, P. (1995). *Alzheimer's disease: Natural feeding techniques.* (1995). [Video]. (Distributed by VA Medical Center, Bedford, MA [617] 687-2936.)

SUGGESTED READING

Hellen, C.R. (1990, March/April). Eating: An Alzheimer's activity. *American Journal of Alzheimer's Care and Related Disorders and Research,* pp. 5–9.

Hellen, C.R. (1992). *Alzheimer's disease: Activity-focused care.* Stoneham, MA: Andover Medical Publishers.

Kovach, C.R. (1997). *Late-stage dementia care: A basic guide.* Washington, DC: Taylor & Francis.

Volicer, L., Seltzer, B., Rheaume, Y., Karner, J., Glennon, M., Riley, M.E., & Crino, P. (1989). Eating difficulties in patients with probable dementia of the Alzheimer type. *Journal of Geriatric Psychiatry and Neurology,* 2(4), 188–195.

Zahler, L., Keiser, A., Gates, G., & Holdt, C. (1994, March/April). Staff attitudes towards the provision of nutritional care to Alzheimer's patients. *American Journal of Alzheimer's Care and Related Disorders and Research,* pp. 31–37.

APPENDIX
LifeStory Book

The caregiving program at the Wealshire [the Wealshire is the author's workplace] includes the compilation of a LifeStory Book, which helps caregivers to get to know new residents before they come to live in the facility. The following letter is sent to residents' families to encourage them to create a LifeStory Book.

Dear Family Member,

The Wealshire is asking for your assistance. As we seek partnership with you in caregiving for your loved one, we wish to know their life story. As you know, the person with dementia often lives in the past, in the "world of work." These years represent a period of time filled with meaningful experiences, many retained as memories. The Wealshire staff wants the opportunity to learn as much as we can about the resident's past so that we can use the information as a basis for our approach to therapeutic caregiving. The LifeStory Book offers the staff insights into likes, dislikes, past interests, and names of key persons and family members. LifeStory information is then adapted for daily interest programs and activities, and it provides opportunities for companionship and reminiscing. The book can be used to help the resident make the often-difficult transition from home to the Wealshire because the staff will "know" the new resident and be capable of building a relationship based on shared memories.

Caregiving at the Wealshire focuses on the residents' remaining abilities. Often, these abilities are enabled and strengthened with information from the resident's LifeStory Book. We hope that you will consider making a book for your loved one.

Making a LifeStory Book

A LifeStory Book can be made from photograph albums, notebooks, or any durable booklet. The Wealshire suggests using a three-ring binder so that pages can be added at any time. Using posterboard or cutting up file folders for paper can provide you with a sturdy page that will survive constant handling. Drawings, writings, pictures, maps, and other visual materials can be used. If you wish to include precious photographs, please photocopy them and keep the original, placing the copy in the LifeStory Book. People with dementia can read for many years, so please write information in short sentences or phrases. Placing names under photographs is especially important. Use a dark pen, printing the words clearly and in large print. The following are suggestions for contents of the LifeStory Book.[2]

Genealogy

Nationality, heritage, birth dates, family tree, siblings, and relationship to resident
Use of short phrases to note important memories about family

---

[2]Adapted from Hellen (1992).

Religious/Spiritual

Background, interest in organized religion
Faith community—pictures of outside, interior, and sanctuary
Current participation
Use of or response to rituals, traditions, blessings, and prayers
Favorite songs and hymns (include words and music)

Personality

Happy? Liked people? Joker? Favorite joke?
Responses to others
Responses to life roles (e.g., father, mother, daughter, son, uncle)
Description of general mood

Childhood/Adolescence

Friends and clubs
Summertime activities
Work history

Education

Grade completed, school names, type of school, degrees
Favorite/least-favorite subjects
Extracurricular activities, sports teams, clubs

Key Life Events

Dates (year), and describe events
Graduations
Marriage, children, dates
Deaths of family members, close friends, important people

Places Lived

Description (map can be included)
Liked/not liked? Why?
Memories of specific rooms, yard, distance from school, shopping
Use of pictures in this section can be evocative

Close Friends, Neighbors

Nature of relationships with friends
Was resident a help to others?

Work History

At home? In the marketplace? Worked alone? Worked with others?

Specific kinds of work and responses to what the resident liked and what he or she did not like about the work

Retirement information

Military History

Of resident, significant family members

Memories of war, peace

Favorite Transportation

Did resident drive? Own a car? What kind?

Use of pictures in this section can be evocative

Awards Received
Clubs, Group Memberships, Leadership Positions

What clubs/groups did resident belong to?

Did resident hold any leadership positions? Describe.

Volunteer Experiences/Service Organizations
Literary Interests

Titles, passages, verses, poetry, scriptures

Recreational Activities/Hobbies
Animals/Pets
Travel

Locations of places visited, favorite places (use maps)

Favorite Foods, Recipes

What were resident's favorite foods?

Liked to cook? Bake? Describe.

Favorite recipes (include copies)

Favorite Holidays, Seasons

Traditions, rituals for each holiday, types of decorations used

Use of pictures in this section can be evocative

Sensory Profile

Resident's Name _____   Date _____

Auditory

Hearing:

Right ear:

Left ear:

___ Adequate

___ Hypersensitive

___ Eyes track to noise
source

___ Distracted from
functional response
by noise

___ Oblivious to noise

Describe response to:

___ Loud noise

___ Unexpected noise

___ Background noise

___ Foreground noise

___ Silence

___ Male voice

___ Female voice

___ Foreign accent

___ Yelling/screaming

Other:

Assistive Devices:

___ Right ear   ___ Left ear

Tolerates devices (describe):

_____

_____

_____

_____

_____

_____

_____

_____

_____

_____

_____

_____

_____

_____

Visual

Vision:

Assistive Devices:

Right eye:

Tolerates devices (describe):

Left eye:

___ Adequate

_____

___ Eyes track to noise
source

_____

___ Squints

_____

___ Eyes closed

_____

___ Avoids eye contact

_____

___ Eye tracks movement

_____

___ Stares

_____

___ Watches others

Figure-ground discrimination: ___ Yes   ___ No

Describe response to:

___ Bright lights

___ Dim lights

___ Blinking lights

___ Darkness

Other:

Gustatory (taste)

___ Hypersensitive

Describe response to:

___ Hyposensitive

___ Sweets

___ Adequate

___ Sour

___ Avoids certain tastes

___ Salty

___ Taste offensive/rejection

___ Rough texture

___ Oral temperature sensitivity

___ Smooth texture

___ Mouths objects/fingers

___ Thin texture

___ Taste discrimination for nonedibles

___ Thick texture

Other:

___ Hot foods, drinks

___ Cold foods, drinks

Olfactory (smell)

___ Adequate

___ Hypersensitive

___ Hyposensitive

Other:

Describe response to:

___ Strong odors

___ Certain smells

___ Pleasant smells

___ Unpleasant smells

Tactile

___ Normal response

___ Hypersensitive

___ Hyposensitive

___ No response

___ Tactile defensive
(specify body part)

___ Touches everything

___ Grabs at others

___ Holds on too tightly

Other:

Describe response to:

___ Standing near others

___ Sitting near others

___ Being messy

___ Grooming/hygiene

___ Water

___ Heat

___ Cold

___ Wind

___ Pain

___ Clothing

Staff Name/Position _____

BEHAVIOR PROFILE

Resident's Name _____

Date _____   Staff Member_____

WHAT
is happening?   Identify and assess
are the resident responses?   Observe: Does the behavior have physical or emotional manifestations or both?

WHERE
is the behavior being exhibited?   Is the behavioral response taking place in a familiar environment?
are there environmental triggers? What are they?

WHEN

does behavior occur?
    Be specific about timing (note time of day, during ADLs?, after family visits?)

Who

is involved?
    Is the behavior a response to a specific person(s)? Caregiver? Family? Visitor?

Why

did the behavior occur?
    Is the behavior really a problem?   Is there poor communication?
    To whom?   What is actually being communicated?
    Is response consistent with   Is the task too complex?
      previous triggers?   Is the behavior an activity?
    Are there medical problems?

What Now

Assistance
Approaches
Changes needed

Interventions (be specific)
   Cognitive
   Physical
   Psychosocial/emotional
   Environmental

Adapted from Hellen (1992).

Behavior Tracking Form

Resident's Name

Date	Time	Observed Activity & Behavior	Behavior			Observer
			Trigger	Intervention	Time Elapsed (before stopping/ stayed stopped)	

FINGER FOODS

When eating utensils escalate anxiety, increase confusion, or lead to the meal not being eaten, utensils can be disregarded totally and eating with fingers commences. Staff concern should not center on good manners versus bad manners. If eating with the fingers allows people with dementia to retain independence during mealtimes, thereby promoting their abilities to be in control and maintain a positive self-image, then the emphasis should shift to finding foods that can be easily grasped, held, and delivered to the mouth, and support their nutritional needs. The following lists comprise suggestions for finger foods. These foods should encourage caregivers to be creative and lead to the development of their own finger-food creations.

BREAKFAST FINGER FOODS

Cereals: small or large shredded wheat, sturdy flakes or cereals with shapes

Eggs: hard boiled; scrambled in chunks, not broken up; scrambled or fried egg sandwiches; deviled eggs

"Take along" biscuit sandwiches with sausage, egg, and cheese

French toast, raisin toast, cinnamon toast

Pancakes

Waffles

Coffee cake, donuts

Peanut butter and jelly sandwiches

Grilled cheese sandwiches

Fruits: all that can be held (dried and fresh) in the hand

LUNCH/SNACK FINGER FOODS

Sandwiches: all kinds that can be held without falling apart using different kinds of breads, rolls, pocket breads (heating sandwiches so the ingredients become sticky helps to keep them together)

Hamburgers, hot dogs

Fruit plates with cheese cubes

Pizza

Salads: all kinds that have pieces big enough to pick up in the hand (e.g., cobb, pasta); roll-up salads using a large lettuce leaf to wrap around ingredients

Fruits: all that can be hand-held, both dried and fresh

Desserts: fruit, cookies, bars, Jell-O cubes, cake, cupcakes, ice cream bars, cones, Popsicles, applesauce cubes made with gelatin

DINNER FINGER FOODS

Meats, poultry, fish, seafood: soft and safe to put in bite-size pieces, nuggets; rolled; placed in sandwiches; cooked into balls, loaves, or pies

Dinner sandwiches: use mashed potatoes to hold in meat and vegetables (toasting bread helps to keep sandwiches from falling apart)

Dinner roll-up: use large cooked cabbage leaf to wrap around meat, vegetable, and rice or potatoes

Quiche pieces: vegetable, meat, seafood

Pasta: use pasta that can be filled with meat or cheese; with or without an extremely thick sauce

Vegetable pieces: carrots, zucchini, cucumbers, tomatoes, Brussels sprouts, celery, beets, beans, corn, green peppers

Potatoes: baked, roasted, French fries, hash browns, oven baked, small boiled

Rolls, biscuits, breads, breadsticks

Cubed jellied cranberry sauce

Pickles, olives

Desserts: fruit, cookies, bars, Jell-O cubes, cake, cupcakes, ice cream bars, cones, Popsicles, applesauce cubes made with gelatin

NUTRIENT-DENSE RECIPES

SUPER PUDDING

2 cups whole milk (cream, heavy cream, or evaporated milk can be substituted for whole milk)
¾ cup dry milk powder
2 tbs vegetable oil
1 package (4½ oz.) instant pudding (select resident's favorite flavor)

Nutrient content per 1-cup serving	
Servings	3
Calories	495
Protein	14 g

Stir together milk, milk powder, and oil in a large bowl. Add instant pudding and mix well. Pour into dishes and refrigerate.

For more calories, use dry milk powder made from whole milk. Serve with cream, heavy cream, whipping cream, vanilla ice cream, or vanilla frozen yogurt.

Recipe courtesy of Carol Johnson, D.T.R.

SUPER CEREAL

Oatmeal, dry	2½ cups
Milk, 2%	⅔ cup
Water	3½ cups
Milk, nonfat dry	1 cup
Margarine	¼ lb
Sugar, brown	½ cup
Sugar, granulated	½ cup

Nutrient content per 8-oz. serving

Servings	4
Calories	564
Protein	13 g
Fat	24 g
Carbohydrates	74 g

Mix water, dry milk, and ⅓ cup of 2% milk. Bring to a boil. Reduce heat to low and pour in oatmeal (or other hot cereal). Cook over low heat until oatmeal is ready (about 5 minutes). Add margarine, sugars, and remaining 2% milk. Cook an additional 5 minutes.

Recipe courtesy of the Wealshire.

14

Management of Occasional and Frequent Problem Behaviors in Dementia

Bathing and Disruptive Vocalization

Philip D. Sloane, M.D., M.P.H., and Ann Louise Barrick, Ph.D.

Alzheimer's disease and related dementias are characterized by disturbances of behavior such as confusion, wandering, repeated questioning, and disorientation. Many of these disturbances are mild and do not cause severe problems for caregivers. Although these problems may be bothersome at home, in institutional settings they tend to be reasonably well tolerated. More severe behavior problems involve manifestations of agitation and aggression that have a significant impact on the lives of others. This chapter provides a framework for thinking about and addressing behavior problems, and provides illustration by examining in detail the management of bathing problems and of disruptive vocalization.

In general, problem behaviors arise because an individual with dementia misinterprets environmental cues (Figure 1). Behavior disorders in dementia can be divided into agitated behaviors and aggressive behaviors. Both agitated and aggressive behaviors can occur in verbal and physical forms (Figure 2). Verbal and physical agitation are the most common forms of disruptive behaviors observed

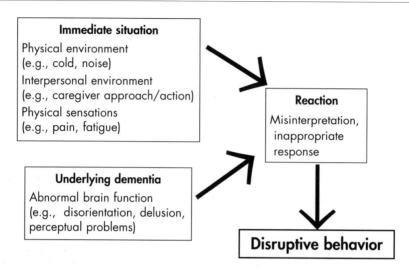

Figure 1.   How brain disease and situational factors interact to cause disruptive behaviors.

in people with dementia. Aggression is much less common than agitation, but tends to be more serious because it poses a physical threat to caregivers and other residents. If caregivers do not address agitated behaviors, the behaviors will progress to aggression; aggression occasionally arises without being preceded by agitation, but this occurrence is unusual. The form of expression (verbal versus physical) of the behavior does not necessarily indicate the severity of the problem. Some individuals, particularly men and people in later stages of dementia, tend to act out physically more readily than others. Women, particularly those with early- and mid-stage dementia, are much more likely to use verbal forms of expression.

	Type of expression	
Severity of expression	Verbal	Physical
Agitation	Common in bathing Common form of disruptive vocalization	Common in bathing
Aggression	Occurs occasionally in bathing Uncommon form of disruptive vocalization	Common in bathing

Figure 2.   Disruptive behaviors in dementia and their relationship to problems in bathing and to disruptive vocalizations.

Define and describe the **P**roblem

Learn about the **P**erson

Brainstorm **P**ossible causes

Develop a **P**lan

If it works, **P**ass it on

Figure 3.   The 5 P's: an approach to problem behaviors in dementia.

Because they express themselves verbally does not necessarily indicate that they are not severely distressed and that the problem should not be addressed.

Agitated behaviors tend to be directed at the environment, whereas aggressive behaviors tend to be directed at individuals. Examples of verbal agitation include yelling, moaning, screaming, and repeating words and phrases such as "help me," all of which are directed into space at no person in particular. Older adults with dementia may demonstrate physical agitation by banging on a tray or table, pacing, or rocking back and forth. Verbally aggressive behaviors may present as swearing at, threatening, or yelling at a staff member or another resident. Examples of physically aggressive behaviors include hitting, biting, kicking, slapping, or spitting at a staff member or another resident. The majority of people with dementia exhibit specific agitated and aggressive behaviors only at specific times. Most individuals who are aggressive are aggressive rarely; most who have severe behavior problems of any type act out only occasionally. The management of disruptive behaviors is dependent on how frequently the behaviors occur: If the behaviors occur occasionally, attention should be directed to the activities or events that precipitate the behaviors. If the behaviors occur frequently, precipitance should be looked for, but a more comprehensive management plan is necessary.

MANAGEMENT OF PROBLEM BEHAVIORS: THE "FIVE P'S"

Staff who are working with older adults with occasional or frequent behavior problems can benefit from a systematic approach—the "five P's"—to their behavior management plan (see also Figure 3):

1.   Define the **problem** behavior. People with dementia who demonstrate disruptive behaviors cannot change; the goal of the behavior management plan is to reduce the incidence of problematic behaviors. The most serious problems staff may experience in bathing a person with dementia are yelling, bit-

ing, or hitting. Identifying the problem is the first step. Once the problem behavior has been identified, staff should discuss when it occurs (e.g., time of day of occurrence is often very telling), to whom it occurs, and how staff respond to it.

2. Learn about the **person** with the problem behavior. In general, the manifestation of disruptive behaviors represents attempts to communicate needs or to express distress. Staff should investigate what triggers cause the person to become anxious or distressed and what provides relief. If the problem behavior occurs during bathing, staff should inquire as to the person's past bathing habits, his or her premorbid attitudes toward bathing, and his or her preferences (e.g., type of soap, bath versus shower, time of day).

3. Brainstorm **possible causes.** Brainstorming is done ideally in a case management conference, which is attended by nursing staff, activities staff, and nursing assistants. Family of the person with dementia should be invited as well. During the meeting, the problem behavior should be identified and discussed, relevant characteristics of the person should be talked about, and the group as a whole should discuss what may be precipitating the behavior (e.g., misinterpretations of the physical environment, pain, delusions, caregivers' behaviors).

4. Develop a management **plan.** The behavior management plan should be comprehensive and should address all of the major causes that were identified. Sometimes a variety of solutions are possible. Solutions should make sense for both staff and resident, should be achievable with current staffing and resources, and should be based on knowledge of the resident and the successes that have been achieved by caregivers and family members. The plan should be implemented, evaluated, and modified based on the responses of all involved in the case. All staff who are involved should be informed about the plan and learn their role(s) in implementing the plan.

5. **Pass** it on. Too often, caregivers learn about techniques that work and then do not tell others. This unfortunate fact is particularly true of nursing assistants, who often develop techniques that effectively manage behavior problems during bathing, dressing, and other activities that involve staff effort. Because, typically, nursing assistants do not communicate extensively with each other or with nurses (a study by the author and colleagues showed that, during an 8-hour workday, nursing assistants spent only 20 minutes talking with other staff members), it takes effort on the part of management to pass on the information. The same is true of a case management plan: Such a plan must be passed on to others in order to be successful.

MANAGEMENT OF OCCASIONAL
BEHAVIOR PROBLEMS: BATHING

> Mr. B. was an 89-year-old man with Alzheimer's disease who resided in a nursing facility. Staff never wanted to bathe him because they knew

he would be difficult. He resisted strenuously the efforts of his caregivers from the moment he was undressed in his room to the end of his bath. During a bath, Mr. B. became increasingly agitated, pulling caregivers' hair and occasionally striking out. He became verbally agitated when his caregivers tried to wash his hair. By the end of the bath, he and staff members were exhausted and he was screaming.

An interdisciplinary case management conference was held to discuss Mr. B's behavior. The caregivers who bathed him met with the nursing staff and a number of issues were discussed:

- Mr. B's agitation began when he was asked to bathe and built gradually so that by the end of the bath, he was yelling and fighting with his bathers. Staff members felt that if the bathing process could be abbreviated, Mr. B. would not become so agitated, and maybe the bath would "go better."
- Mr. B. seemed threatened by his caregivers; he is a private man.
- A particular problem was washing Mr. B's hair because, often, soap ran into his eyes. Also, he had severe arthritis, and staff noted that any movement of his legs, toes, and arms made him scream or hit.
- Although Mr. B. was not very verbal, often, at the end of a bath, he complained of being cold.

In response to these issues, attendees of the case management conference developed a comprehensive treatment plan for Mr. B. He was to receive two acetaminophen tablets for his arthritis pain as soon as he got up in the morning. Then he was to be wheeled to the bathing area, his pajamas removed, and he and the chair placed in the shower. A male caregiver (preferable because of Mr. B's private nature) was to assist him, providing eye contact, a reassuring manner, continuing conversation about things of interest to Mr. B. (e.g., fishing, trucks), and an explanation of what he was doing before he did it. The caregiver found that, by being patient, he could involve Mr. B. in washing his own genitals, thus alleviating one of his sources of embarrassment. He also found that Mr. B's hair could be washed without water getting in his eyes if he tilted Mr. B's head back and held a washcloth over his forehead. When the bath was completed, a large cotton blanket was wrapped around Mr. B. and a towel was placed over his head to keep him warm. With these measures, disruptive behaviors were almost eliminated in Mr. B.

APPROACHES TO COMMON BEHAVIOR PROBLEMS IN BATHING

Solving the behavior problems of people with dementia during bathing requires staff to take an individualized, psychosocial approach, such as the five P's. An individualized, psychosocial approach is focused on the older adult's needs, likes, dislikes, history, and remaining cognitive abilities. Often, the focus in bathing is on cleaning up the person as quickly as possible, which can easily result in the older adult becoming agitated, aggressive, or both. When problem behaviors manifest themselves, it is important for the caregiver to stop and systematically assess the situation. The steps involved in such an assessment include determining the goal of the bath; describing the problem behaviors; understanding the person; discovering the possible causes, or triggers; and developing strategies for decreasing the problem behaviors and preserving the person's privacy and dignity. Specific factors related to each step follow.

STEP 1: DESCRIBE THE PROBLEM BEHAVIOR

Caregivers should observe the behavior of the person with dementia carefully and identify specific problems. In doing so, they should gather as much information as possible about who is involved or present when the behavior problem(s) occur, what the problem(s) are, where the problem(s) occur, and when the problem(s) occurs. Other factors that should be considered are what takes place before and after the behavior problem occurs and what intervention seems to be successful in calming the person.

STEP 2: UNDERSTAND THE PERSON WITH PROBLEM BEHAVIOR

A variety of personal information can help solve behavior problems. Important information that caregivers can use to reduce problem behaviors includes knowing the individual's level of dementia, any physical problems he or she has, and his or her personal history. Staff should use different types of interventions, depending on the person's level of dementia. For example, the milder the dementia, the more useful are the techniques of conversing, encouraging independence, and making choices. Physical distractions such as chewing gum or providing something to hold and postponing tasks are more effective interventions for people in later stages of dementia.

Knowledge of the individual's physical problems is important because some disruptive behavior in bathing stems from an inability to communicate physical pain clearly. If the person experiences pain from such conditions as arthritis, extra care may need to be taken when washing the painful area. If the person's mobility is poor, a lift may be needed. Staff should check for areas on the skin that are sensitive and for any treatable illnesses.

Knowledge of the person's premorbid occupation and hobbies, family members and friends who are important to the person, cultural background, special qualities and abilities, and his or her likes and dislikes can help caregivers to better understand problem behavior and develop an individualized, appropriate intervention plan. Other important factors in a personal history with which staff should become conversant are the person's preferences for time of day to bathe, the type of bath (e.g., tub, shower), and gender of caregiver.

STEP 3: LOOK FOR POSSIBLE TRIGGERS FOR THE PROBLEM BEHAVIOR

Often, incidents of problem behavior are generated by certain triggers. Possible triggers include the person's level of dementia, any physical problems he or she may have, the environment, the caregiving procedure itself, and the manner in which the caregiver communicates with the person with dementia. Caregivers must pay attention to these triggers and amend caregiving procedures accordingly. The following questions can be used by staff as guidelines for reducing disruptive behaviors in the older adults for whom they care and for amending their caregiving techniques so that they are appropriate to the individual:

- Level of dementia: What are the communication abilities of the individual? Does he or she have difficulty with impulse control, judgment, or misunderstanding? Is he or she unable to tell staff what is wrong?
- Physical problems: Is the person in pain, tired, depressed, constipated, or on too much medication/medications that have adverse interactions? Does the person have a hearing or visual impairment?
- Environment: Is the environment too noisy, too new/unfamiliar, too crowded, too bright, or too cold or hot for the person?
- Caregiving procedure: Is the caregiving procedure too complex and confusing, unfamiliar, or too fast for the person? Are there too many caregivers?
- Communication technique: Do caregivers speak too fast and/or use complex sentences? Is a friendly, calm approach with good eye contact used in bathing the person? Is each step explained?

STEP 4: DEVELOP A PLAN

Once the likely causative factors have been cataloged and examined, a comprehensive, effective behavior management plan should be developed. The first step of the plan is to examine critically the goals of the bath. Many residents of nursing facilities are scheduled for two to three baths a week. When bathing or the prospect of bathing causes a resident to become distressed, staff should ask themselves whether this bath is necessary: Does the resident have an infection control or social issue that needs to be addressed? For example, does he or she have a skin infection or pustule, or is there an unpleasant skin odor? If so, a bath may be necessary; if not, it may be best to postpone the bath to make the experience as stress-free as possible. Also, caregivers may need to consider postponing some tasks, giving a partial bath, or using a no-rinse body shampoo in order to guard against possible agitation or aggression.

In developing an effective behavior management plan, it is best to meet with all caregivers, including family members. The discussion should revolve around the behavior problem, its causes, and possible interventions. The interventions that are developed should be implemented one at a time and each given a fair trial. The intervention should be changed as needed to emphasize what works and eliminate strategies that are not useful. Staff also should remember that each bath should be individualized or tailored to the person's needs, preferences and abilities, and specific behavior problem. Some other general guidelines include the following:

- Focus more attention on the person than on the task—Although getting a person clean is important, a "car-wash approach" to bathing may cause both older adult and caregiver discomfort.
- Be flexible—Be open to making changes in the plan. Alter the caregiving approach (e.g., do not use the word "bath"), alter the procedure (e.g., instead of washing the person's hair at the beginning of the bath, do it later), or alter the environment (e.g., try a bed bath).
- Use persuasion, not coercion—Let the person feel that he or she is in control, provide the person with opportunities to make choices, and encourage independence as much as possible. Use distractions and take shortcuts in bathing when possible. Respond positively to the person and praise him or her sincerely and often. Always use a reassuring, supportive style during the bath.
- Stop—When a person becomes agitated, stop, assess the situation, and use a behavior management technique that is included in the person's individualized plan to prevent problem behaviors from escalating.
- Ask for help—Talking with others about challenges faced in bathing the person gives staff an opportunity to brainstorm other solutions that have not been tried.

MANAGEMENT OF FREQUENT
BEHAVIOR PROBLEMS: DISRUPTIVE VOCALIZATIONS

Mrs. H. was a 79-year-old woman with multi-infarct dementia living in a nursing facility. She had had several strokes and used a wheelchair. Her disruptive vocalizations had increased over several months. She made statements such as "help me!" and "Curtis is going to kill my baby!" commonly. Typically, she yelled during and after dressing, and following lunch, she yelled almost continuously until dinner. Facility staff found that Mrs. H's vocalizations ceased with one-to-one attention, but the staffing situation was such that they could not provide her with as much individual attention as she needed. Staff also found that Haldol was helpful, but only in doses high enough to put her to sleep. At night, Mrs. H. was reported to be relatively quiet.

An interdisciplinary case management conference was held, with Mrs. H's family present. It was found that Mrs. H. had a long history of depression. It was also discovered that Curtis was her common-law husband, with whom she lived during her 20s and 30s and who was known to be physically abusive. Conferees felt that Mrs. H. probably experienced some discomfort as a result of being nonambulatory; and that her vocalizations increased when she became incontinent.

A management plan was developed for Mrs. H. The plan included administration of an antidepressant, to which she responded well. In addition, because it was felt that her vocalization probably represented a combination of anxiety and disinhibition, attempts were made to provide interventions that would decrease her anxiety or otherwise occupy her. Staff were given the following options to employ when Mrs. H. began to vocalize:

- Provide Mrs. H. with soothing audiotapes of a human heartbeat, the ocean, and new age music that she can listen to on a portable stereo.
- Check Mrs. H's incontinence pad to see if it needs to be changed. Offer her food and drink.
- Offer one-to-one attention, with reassurance and, if needed, relocation (e.g., to the patio).

Staff felt empowered because they had several interventions available to them and because they understood Mrs. H's problems better. The combination therapies did not cause her disruptive vocalizations to cease altogether, but they became much less prolonged. Thus, everyone on the interdisciplinary team felt that the behavior management plan was a success.

MANAGEMENT APPROACH TO THE OLDER ADULT WITH DISRUPTIVE VOCALIZATIONS

In behaviors that occur frequently, precipitants should be looked for, but a comprehensive behavior management plan is necessary. Management of the older adult with disruptive vocalizations involves four steps: define the problem by describing the behavior, learn about the person through medical evaluation and family interviews, identify causes and triggers, and develop a management plan.

STEP 1: DEFINE THE PROBLEM BY DESCRIBING THE BEHAVIOR

Staff should be aware that some vocalizations are intermittent and occur only in certain situations; other vocalizations occur frequently. Some vocalizations are relatively quiet, whereas others are extremely loud. Using these guidelines, staff should describe who is involved or present when the vocalizations occur; what the vocalizations are; where the vocalizations occur; when the vocalizations occur; the loudness, frequency, and timing of the vocalization(s); whether any nonverbal activities (e.g., pacing, banging on tables, throwing things) were associated with the vocalization; and how staff and other residents responded.

STEP 2: LEARN ABOUT THE PERSON THROUGH MEDICAL EVALUATION AND FAMILY INTERVIEWS

A medical evaluation should be conducted to evaluate the cognitive status, psychiatric status, and physical status of the individual with dementia. Evaluating the person's cognitive status is important because, in general, people with mild or moderate dementia respond to interpersonal interventions such as activities, whereas people with end-stage dementia tend to respond to one-to-one care or physical interventions such as audiotapes, a teddy bear, or aromatherapy. The clinician conducting the physical examination should look for emergent neurological disease or other medical problems (e.g., constipation, urinary tract infection), treatable sensory impairment (e.g., cataracts), sources of pain and discomfort (e.g., undetected fractures, arthritis), delusions or mood disorders (e.g., depression), and complications of immobility (e.g., contractures).

The family interview gives staff an opportunity to learn from family members clues as to what underlies the anxiety or other emotional state of the person with dementia. Family members may give information about names and events that the person mentions in the vocalizations. In addition, a history of prior psychiatric disease or prior losses, abuse, and stress is often expressed by family.

STEP 3: IDENTIFY CAUSES AND TRIGGERS

One key to understanding the cause of disruptive vocalization is to listen for the message the resident is expressing. For example, "leave me alone," often indicates overstimulation. Similarly, statements such as "you're going to kill me," indicate extremely abnormal, often psychotic perceptions. Expressions such as "help me," or "oh, my God!" are generally manifestations of anxiety. Vocalizations such as "na-na-na-na-na" often occur in individuals who have poor hearing and vision and who are sensorily deprived.

Also, identify triggers that aggravate or induce the behavior. Triggers can include factors related to the individual such as sensory deprivation, psychological distress, discomfort/pain, and fatigue; factors related to the external environment such as overstimulation, understimulation, noise, or glare; and caregiver behaviors such as restriction of freedom, a harsh approach, or rough handling of the person.

STEP 4: DEVELOP A PLAN

In identifying what relieves the behavior, staff are often the most helpful source because they have noted a variety of solutions to the vocalization. An interdisciplinary case management conference is the best method of identifying these effective interventions. Once possible causes have been listed, other solutions should be brainstormed. Some of the solutions include the following:

- Measures to reduce overstimulation (e.g., avoiding large-group activities, the dining area)
- Measures to decrease sensory deprivation and understimulation (e.g., involvement in social activities, location near a high-traffic area, the use of music)
- Treatment of pain and discomfort with medication
- Reduction of the loss of freedom that results from immobility by taking the people outdoors, wheeling them about, positioning them in an area of choice, or removing physical restraints, and minimizing fatigue by reducing overstimulation, controlling the length of activities and visits, and scheduling regular naps

The management plan should address the causes of the disruptive vocalization, be comprehensive, and provide staff with a "tool kit" of modalities that everyone wants to try in different situations. In developing the plan it should be emphasized to staff that all vocalizations arise for a reason and that the vocalizer is *distressed* rather than *distressing*. Caregivers must be reminded not to overreact to the vocalization. Indeed, the vocalization may be good for the individual's health because it provides the lungs with exercise. The plan encourages staff to recognize that change will occur—most disruptive vocalizers either improve or become sicker. Many have end-stage Alzheimer's disease. Staff should be sympathetic, tolerant, and energetic in trying to relieve the individual's distress.

CONCLUSION

Alzheimer's disease is primarily a behavioral disease. To solve problem behaviors, caregivers must be detectives and seek to understand what the person with dementia is experiencing. A systematic approach such as the five P's should be employed as a solution.

SUGGESTED READING

Burgio, L., Flynn, W., & Martin, D. (1987). Disruptive vocalization in institutionalized geriatric patients. *Gerontologist, 27,* 285.

Burgio, L., Scilley, K., Hardin, J., Janosky, J., Bonino, P., Slater, S., & Engberg, R. (1994). Studying disruptive vocalization and contextual factors in the nursing home using computer-assisted real-time observation. *Journal of Gerontology, 49*(5), 230–239.

Cohen-Mansfield, J., Werner, P., & Marx, M. (1990). Screaming in nursing home residents. *Journal of the American Geriatrics Society, 38*(7), 755–792.

Rader, J. (1994). To bathe or not to bathe: That is the question. *Journal of Gerontological Nursing, 20*(9), 53–54.

Sloane, P., Honn, V., Dwyer, S., Wieselquist, J., & Cain, C. (1995). Bathing the Alzheimer's patient in long term care: Results and recommendations from three studies. *American Journal of Alzheimer's Disease, 10*(4), 3–8.

Sloane, P., Rader, J., Barrick, A., Hoeffer, B., Dwyer, S., McKenzie, D., Lavelle, M., Buckwalter, K., Arrington, L., & Pruitt, T. (1995). Bathing persons with dementia. *Gerontologist, 35*(5), 672–678.

15

Sexuality, Intimacy, and Meaningful Relationships in the Nursing Facility

Staff and Family Roles in the Care of People with Alzheimer's Disease

Edna L. Ballard, M.S.W., A.C.S.W.

Something wonderful has happened! A love affair! Yes, the new man in his eighties, a retired eye doctor, and the former Berkeley professor! He insists he wants to "lie down to rest" with her in her bed. Some of the staff is pleased; it's the first time I've seen any real life happening in the Manor. Some nurses think it's a nuisance and a hazard. Their children are against it. But for once, Maury and I agree. We both wish the woman were Ma.

—Elaine Marcus Starkman, 1993

Studies indicate that the majority of physically healthy men and women in the presence of a willing and able partner remain sexually active on a regular basis, even into the eighth or ninth decade (e.g., Kaplan, 1991). As the result of such studies, conventional attitudes and beliefs are less rigid in the supposition that older people are not interested in sexual activity (George & Weiler, 1981; Starr, 1985). However, older individuals who can no longer live independently; who need help with self-care tasks such as dressing, maintaining personal hygiene, toileting, and feeding themselves; and whose cognitive ability is compromised often are not viewed or treated as sexual beings. Dependence becomes equated with asexuality; the more dependent and impaired the individual, the less credence is given to sexual or intimacy needs. The mission of the nursing facility staff, the facility administration, and the family becomes one of protecting the individual from self and others in sexual matters. Residents who do not conform to this expectation and who express behaviors with sexual overtones are often labeled "disinhibited" and "disruptive" to the nursing facility environment. All too often, the personal needs-oriented perspective of the resident is sacrificed to appeasing family members who may object, a fear of legal repercussions, unresolved ethical questions, or a focus on bureaucratic policies and efficient routines (Ballard, 1996). Policies and procedures, written and unwritten, are rigidly enforced in most nursing care facilities in order to control the sexual behaviors of residents. Nevertheless, the individual with Alzheimer's disease remains a sexual being.

Sexuality and intimacy are important aspects of the life of every human being. Individuals, of course, vary in their interest and sexual activity. Many individuals live full and satisfying lives without physical sexual activity; others characterize the quality of their lives by the presence or absence of sexual activity with another individual(s) or view the sexual aspect of the marriage or relationship as integral to the fulfillment of that relationship. Alzheimer's disease and related dementias can bring about dramatic changes in personality and behavior, including sexual interest and behaviors. As Alzheimer's disease progresses, people with the disease generally experience diminished sexual interest and activity. Moreover, as the disease progresses, people with Alzheimer's disease are likely to become self-centered, indifferent to the needs of others, unaware of the consequences of their actions, and unable to fulfill their expected role in the relationship. Still, being treated with warmth, affection, and respect; being touched; and having the opportunity to touch others remain important to the well-being of the older adult, even in late stages of the dementing illness. Families and professionals who care for people with Alzheimer's disease are required to respond appropriately to them as they are changed by the disease.

WHEN BEHAVIOR BECOMES "PROBLEM" BEHAVIOR

Sexual behavior and interest become problematic when they are viewed as inappropriate or hazardous to the individual involved or to others. Disturbing behaviors, whether agitation, wandering, catastrophic reactions, or inappropriate sexual behaviors, occur, most often, because the resident does not understand what is expected of him or her. Simple requests may seem too complex. The individual feels threatened, confused, and abandoned. The increasing loss of memory affects judgment in making decisions. The individual who is confused or frightened may shadow or cling to staff and attempt to find comfort or reassurance in physical behaviors that may be viewed as sexual and inappropriate. Holding hands, kissing, hugging, self-stimulation, exposing oneself during personal care tasks, and so forth may be an attempt to find meaning and security in an environment that now seems unsafe, unfamiliar, and confusing. As defined by others, "sexual behaviors" may not have a sexual meaning for the resident who, because of impaired judgment or memory, undresses in public or fondles himself or herself for reasons other than sexual gratification. As such, these behaviors require the same careful assessment, evaluation, and care plan as do other behavioral symptoms.

Staff and family each have a role in creating a therapeutic environment for people with Alzheimer's disease. With the progressive loss of memory, confusion, and inability to reason and make decisions, people benefit from increased attention to environments that provide for their total well-being. A therapeutic environment, defined as including people, activities, routines, and stimuli that influence how residents feel and behave, can help people with Alzheimer's disease continue functioning and enjoying life to their highest potential: "All aspects of the person's daily life are either therapeutic or nontherapeutic. The person will need help to become engaged in activities which are meaningful, rewarding, give pleasure and offer opportunities for mastery" (Alzheimer's Association, 1992, p. 24). A therapeutic environment also supports the opportunity for companionship; friendship; and where, when, and for whom appropriate, sexual intimacy. Burger, Fraser, Hunt, and Frank (1996) suggest that good care in the nursing facility includes creating a psychologically secure and physically safe space for residents based on their needs and accommodating as much as possible preferences in such areas as activities of daily living, habits, and past activities. This accommodation helps residents to retain some thread of continuity to their past, which is helpful in forging new relationships and new roles for themselves. The care plan should be specific, individualized, easy to understand, and written so that it can be monitored and evaluated on an ongoing basis as their condition and needs change.

CHALLENGING RESIDENT SEXUAL BEHAVIORS FACED BY NURSING FACILITY STAFF

Many factors influence the number and kind of sexual problems in a nursing facility, including how the problem is defined and viewed, the attitude and training of staff, the size and population mix of the facility, and the unique characteristics and behaviors of individual residents. The staff and administration may respond with a well-considered protocol and specific techniques for handling sexual situations or respond, as one staff member put it, "as quietly as possible, hoping the resident will forget about it."

Following a training seminar requested by the 21 regional North Carolina Ombudsmen responsible for resolving resident and/or family questions and concerns and for ensuring the rights of residents in nursing facilities, the Ombudsmen were surveyed informally on issues about sexual behavior problems in the facilities for which they were responsible (see the appendix at the end of the chapter). Of the nine who responded, eight stated that increased discussion is an area requiring urgent attention. It is important to note that sexual behavior problems in nursing facilities are not so much a matter of frequency but of intensity of staff and family response; tensions and concerns are heightened because of the nature of the problem and the lack of consensus about management approaches. Families become frustrated, embarrassed, and angry, and spouses, in particular, may experience feelings of betrayal. Often, staff are inconsistent in their responses and care strategies. In response to the survey question, "how many situations regarding problems of a sexual nature have you encountered during the course of your career?," the Ombudsmen reported an average of 8, ranging from a high of 30 incidents to 0 incidents. The majority of the respondents reported feeling inadequate and unprepared to handle sexual problems and felt that they were particularly lacking in knowledge regarding residents' right to consent, residents' privacy rights, and appropriate staff responses. When asked to "briefly describe a challenging sexual concern you have confronted in a nursing facility in the past," and asked, "how was the above problem resolved?", respondents included the following examples:

A husband without cognitive impairment and his wife with dementia, both residents in the facility, were having intercourse. The facility staff were not sure that the wife was competent to give reasoned consent. The adult children were concerned as well, but were somewhat reassured that their mother still recognized their father.

Resolution: Staff intervened to end the activity. The wife's behavior changed negatively when these conjugal visits were interrupted by staff, so they were allowed to continue.

A man with mild dementia has sexually fondled female residents in advanced stages of dementia. Despite repeated talks with the man, he repeats the behavior and denies that he has done anything improper.

Resolution: To date, his problem behavior continues. The Ombudsman assigned to the nursing facility set up a meeting with the resident to get to know him and to give him the opportunity for appropriate social interaction. He is also scheduled for a mental health assessment. (*Note:* The respondent stated that problems of a sexual nature in this facility are resolved typically with threats of legal action against the resident in question and/or threats of discharge.)

A male resident was threatened with discharge from the facility for inappropriate sexual behaviors toward female residents. Staff members have made no attempt to involve the resident in activities, find ways to divert or distract him, or develop appropriate ways to hug or provide needed human contact.

Resolution: A care plan was developed for this individual, which included building self-esteem and providing affection and attention. Staff was educated about the effects of Alzheimer's disease and residents' continuing need for human contact. Medications were increased initially and then decreased gradually. (*Note:* The respondent reported that medications, physical restraints, or the threat of discharge may be the first consideration when staff feel threatened by inappropriate behavior and have not been instructed in how to respond in ways that make a positive difference.)

A male resident grabbed the 7-year-old daughter of a resident's visiting family member and asked for sexual favors.

Resolution: After the resident committed repeated aggressive sexual offenses and made verbal threats, he was placed in a state psychiatric hospital.

Two residents with dementia were involved in an interracial relationship; both were married to other people and their families were unaware of the relationship.

Resolution: One resident became ill, so the relationship resolved itself. (*Note:* The respondent reported that in this facility such problems are resolved typically by changing rooms, ignoring or embarrassing the people involved, administering medications, applying restrictive clothing, or requesting a mental health assessment from an independent agency. This challenging problem was viewed as a care management and moral issue by the respondent. Suggested areas for discussion and training included interracial relationships, sexual preferences, competency of one or both partners, and commitment [i.e., pursuing a sexual relationship with a resident when the spouse lives in the community].)

Respondents to the questionnaire suggested the following additional topics for a training curriculum: sexuality and aging; issue of privacy as a right; how to cope with inappropriate aggression in people with head injury; how to prevent inappropriate sexual behaviors and specific diversion techniques; and therapeutic ways to provide affection, intimacy, and an increased sense of well-being for activity directors, floor staff, and others caring for the person with dementia who acts out sexually. In general, people responding to the survey, other nursing facility staff, social workers, and other professionals and family members express a sense of frustration and helplessness in handling a problem that is emotionally taxing and that presents a management crisis when there is a lack of training or skills, protocol, or general consensus on what is the appropriate action and what is in the best interest of the people involved, as in the following case study:

> Mrs. C.[1] had become an embarrassment to her family and to the nursing facility where she had lived for the past 2 months. Her two daughters, son, and only sister began visiting her less often because of her indiscriminate sexual activity. A few "eyebrow-raising incidents" occurred several weeks prior to her placement, but this new, aggressive behavior was unlike anything the family had observed. She made

---

[1] Case example courtesy of Cornelia Poer, M.S.W., A.C.S.W., Social Work Consultant, Durham, NC. Used with permission.

increasingly overt sexual overtures to staff, visitors, and other residents. She could be found frequently in various stages of undress or in a male resident's room. The family was frightened, frustrated, and saddened. Staff tried a series of interventions (e.g., distraction, closer monitoring of her activities, massage therapy to provide attention and comfort), but nothing seemed to work. The family was advised to begin looking for a "more appropriate" facility for Mrs. C. unless there was a significant change in her behavior.

In the case of Mrs. C., staff also tried food as distraction, aromatherapy to provide comfort and attention, and late-afternoon walks in the sunshine, but these too had little effect on reducing the unwanted behaviors. In addition, they counseled other staff who had contact with Mrs. C. on how to best respond to her sexual advances. Mrs. C. was initially diagnosed as hypersexual. This diagnosis limited the options for staff because the overall goal became one of containment. Kuhn, Greiner, and Arsenault (in press) define hypersexuality as persistent sexual behaviors that may range from flirtation to aggressive initiation of sexual activity, which may be directed at one or more people. Behavior that may be observed as hypersexuality, particularly in residents, may be defined as normal and appropriate outside the long-term care setting. Moreover, persistent behavior that may represent a bid for attention, reassurance, acceptance, or some other unmet need may be labeled as hypersexuality. Defining behavior and developing management and care techniques to address it are difficult. The problem is compounded further by clinicians and staff who differ widely on what is acceptable and appropriate behavior in people with dementia. In addition, residents respond differently to different interventions. Simply allowing frightened, depressed residents who need simple reassurance and comfort sufficient time to adjust to living in the facility may be the most relevant intervention. Other older adults may need a variety of management techniques, including medication, applied over a period of time in order to control the behavior.

Research and practice provide little in the way of guidelines for the use of medications to control hypersexuality in people with dementia. Although there is no conclusive evidence regarding the efficacy of drugs (e.g., antipsychotics, antidepressants, anxiolytics, beta blockers, lithium, anticonvulsants) used to treat agitation in dementia, they are sometimes prescribed to treat hypersexuality, particularly when accompanied by agitation or aggression (Kuhn, Greiner, & Arsenault, in press). Clinical reports suggest success in a small percentage of cases. However, there are no controlled studies to clarify under what conditions or which drugs would be useful in the treatment of hypersexuality in people with dementia. Nonpharmacologic behavioral interventions such as addressing the emotional, self-esteem needs of the individual, controlling or eliminating triggers to undesirable behaviors, or manipulating the environment to influence behaviors continue to be viable means of responding to these behaviors.

- *When is staff intervention required?*

  Is this the appropriate place?

  Do both participants have the capacity to consent?

  Is there a potential for harm or injury?

  Is there a third party, such as a spouse or partner in the community who objects to the behavior?

- *What are the appropriate, available options for specific sexual behaviors?*

  Support behavior (e.g., provision of privacy, therapeutic support, information)?

  Distraction, when and where the behavior is inappropriate or harmful?

  Substitution (e.g., providing other ways to meet the affection, self-esteem, sexual needs of residents)?

- *Is this the correct response for this situation?*

  What objective is being met?

- *What are the measures of success?*

  Whose needs are being met?

Figure 1.   Key questions to ask when responding to sexually charged situations. (From Ballard, E.L. [1996]. Sexuality in the special care unit. In S.B. Hoffman & M. Kaplan [Eds.], *Special care programs for people with dementia.* Health Professions Press, Baltimore. With permission.)

STAFF RESPONSES TO RESIDENTS' SEXUAL BEHAVIORS

People with Alzheimer's disease or other dementias may be unable to discriminate as to which people or places are appropriate to express or initiate intimate behavior—behavior that is a legitimate need and a right of the individual and yet may be disruptive to the nursing facility environment. The dilemma for staff becomes how to manage that behavior and within what constraints and limitations. Responses may range from ignoring the behavior to lobbying for discharge of the person(s). Staff reactions to residents' sexual behaviors are determined by the individual staff member's beliefs, fears, and concerns about aging in general and about the caregiver's responsibility to people with dementia. Most often, these reactions are a reflection of how the larger society views sexual expression in older, dependent people. Although attitudes are changing, many responses (e.g., anger, disgust, embarrassment, rejection, derision, ridicule, fear) remain rooted in old beliefs, laws including religious doctrine, attitudes, and traditions.

Training and the opportunity to discuss concerns provide staff with a framework for evaluating behaviors objectively and choosing useful methods of responding (Figure 1 provides a basic, useful response tool). Training eliminates the tendency to ignore or repress the behavior and instead tends to engender a search for more effective ways to help residents meet a legitimate need. Behavior previously defined as problematic often is redefined or rendered moot when viewed objectively. When staff gain understanding and skills in managing difficult behaviors, they are empowered to act confidently and effectively, and this attitude is conveyed to their residents (Hoffman, Platt, & Barry, 1987). Their empowerment serves them not only in difficult situations such as coping with residents' agitation and combativeness but also in care situations that involve sexual behaviors.

KEY ASSUMPTIONS ABOUT RESIDENTS' SEXUALITY IN PLANNING THEIR CARE

The following assumptions about sexuality are basic to providing resident care (Ballard & Poer, 1993):

- All individuals are sexual beings beginning at birth and continuing throughout the life span.
- Even the most impaired, dependent people with dementia retain adult feelings and should be treated as adults.
- Most people with dementia respond to the opportunity to give and receive affection, and to interact with other individuals on various social and emotional levels.
- People with dementia may express inappropriate sexual behaviors because they cannot remember or understand the consequences or meaning of such behaviors.
- Behaviors may appear sexual when there is no sexual meaning for the individual executing the behavior (e.g., disrobing because of discomfort or the need to go to the bathroom, fondling oneself out of boredom or understimulation).
- Staff may reinforce unwanted or inappropriate behaviors by overreacting or by gesture, behavior, or manner of communicating with residents.
- Staff training determines how well residents' needs are met. Attitudes, values, and biases have a direct impact on how staff respond to sexual issues and behaviors and determine the kinds of interventions or management techniques chosen.

OPTIONS FOR RESIDENT CARE AND BEHAVIOR MANAGEMENT

Nursing facility staff who work with residents who are sexually expressive benefit from training by demonstrating an increased confidence in responding to sexual behaviors (Ballard, 1996; Malatesta, 1989; Smith, 1995). Training should provide concrete approaches to supporting residents in meeting legitimate intimacy needs in positive, dignified ways that are acceptable to the resident, family, and staff. Individuals who become proficient in responding to the sexual behaviors of people with dementia must first become personally and professionally comfortable with their own sexuality and views on aging (Malatesta, 1989). Historically, issues of sex and intimacy have been neglected and taboo topics in long-term care facilities. The nursing facility that has a clear protocol for dealing with crises involving resident autonomy, ethical questions, resident safety in sexual matters, and family concerns about sexual issues is likely to resolve sexually charged situations in the best interest of all involved. Without training, staff members are more likely to view expressions of intimacy and sexuality as a nuisance and a hazard, and their role becomes that of extinguishing the behavior at all costs. Under these circumstances the facility may provide competent care at the expense of compassionate care—care that goes beyond the goal of a clean, safe environment and responds to the social, emotional, spiritual, and intimacy needs of residents.

Of course, there are hazards in active sexual behaviors in the nursing facility that must be given careful consideration:

- Medical/physical hazards (e.g., sexually transmitted diseases, exacerbation of concurrent medical problems, potential injury from sexual activity)
- Exploitation of the partner, which may occur even with the consent of this individual
- Harm or distress caused to family or others by the behavior
- Responsibility to staff and other residents may not be met (e.g., behaviors that are considered private and appropriate in one setting may become public and inappropriate in the long-term care setting)
- Legal consequences (e.g., failure to protect vulnerable individual, issues of right to choose versus capacity to consent)
- Ethical considerations (i.e., issues of moral responsibility to resident and others)

RESIDENT-SPECIFIC GOALS FOR DESIGNING CARE

At the heart of designing a care and behavior management program that addresses the sexual interests and behaviors of nursing facility residents are questions about goals for the resident. The resident-specific goals listed here are central to effecting care plans that encompass the physical, emotional, spiritual, and sexual needs of the individual with dementia:

- Build self-esteem by paying special attention to "failure-free environments," which ensure success without being demeaning or condescending.
- Build residents' self-respect; they should not be made to feel less valued because of their diminished skills and abilities. People with Alzheimer's dis-

ease may express their frustration with statements such as, "I am just a big dummy," or "I can't do anything anymore."

- Plan activities and structure the environment to help residents develop interpersonal relationships that increase their sense of community and act as a buffer against loneliness and isolation.
- Maximize functional abilities by allowing residents to continue to do as many self-care tasks as they can manage without regard to how long it takes or how well it is done.
- Support remaining skills and find ways of providing opportunities for success.
- Provide residents with the opportunity to be useful, to contribute to the nursing facility community.
- Promote security in a predictable, supportive, but nondemanding environment.
- Accept unique personality characteristics and behaviors that define the individual.
- Build a caring atmosphere in which residents learn to trust staff.
- Support family involvement with the resident; provide specific guidelines, education, and resources to increase their knowledge of ways to support the resident in the facility.

INTIMACY AND THE NEED TO RESTORE A SENSE OF BELONGING IN NEWLY ADMITTED RESIDENTS

It is neither uncommon nor unexpected that adjustment in the initial phase of nursing facility placement produces feelings of anxiety, fear, confusion, anger, and, sometimes, homelessness. The transition from the community to a nursing facility is traumatic for most people and may be particularly heightened in the person with cognitive impairment. Nursing facility placement is an immediate and often absolute loss of privacy, choice, and autonomy in making decisions about basic life events and activities. It is a loss of people, places, and "things" that may have provided a connection critical to knowing who one is, one's normative role, and what one can expect of others and what others expect of him or her. Although placement can and does engender a measure of security and safety for some individuals, others experience losses and changes that undermine feelings of security and safety in the initial phases of adjustment. It is the search for security, connectedness, and a sense of belonging that may be at the root of some unwanted or inappropriate behaviors. "It is by our roles that we identify ourselves and often it is for our roles we feel loved and valued" (Mace, 1987, p. 16).

Residents' sense of belonging can be restored and maintained when they are treated with dignity and respect and are given consideration as adults. Too often, people with dementia are discounted and treated as though they are invisible because they are no longer capable of fulfilling previous roles. People with dementia who retain some insight into their losses complain that professionals and sometimes even family members will talk about them as if they are not present; become impatient when they take too long to respond to a question or complete a task; or "take over," leaving the person feeling that he has been relegated unnecessarily and prematurely to a "sick role." All of this leaves the individual feeling more inadequate; less like an adult; and less deserving of adult privileges, needs, and rights. Sarah Vann Wyne, a research analyst with the Duke University Neurological Disorders Clinic and facilitator to a support group for people with Alzheimer's disease and their spouses, offers the following reminders from people in the support group about what it is like to have Alzheimer's disease and how others can help them:

"I am not less of a person because I have Alzheimer's disease."

"I am what I am and that's all that I am. I think of myself as normal."

"Consideration! Be considerate of me and my feelings. I still have feelings!"

"Please don't ignore me as though I don't exist. I am a human being. I am not invisible."

"Be tolerant of me, but don't tolerate me."

"Let me do what I can. Give me a try."

It is understandable that the individual who has no idea why he is in the nursing facility responds with anger, fear, depression, or confusion when he seeks to create or define new roles within the limitations of the disease: "The (person) with Alzheimer's disease is in a giant classroom every day, one in which he or she never has the exact answer" (Bell & Troxel, 1997, p. 17). The person with dementia is particularly vulnerable at this stage; nursing facility staff and family members must be acutely attuned to what the resident needs to adjust to his or her new environment. Many factors influence how the resident may respond (Gwyther, 1997):

Physical causes

    Illness, medication, pain

    Hearing or vision loss

    Constipation, dehydration

    Fatigue, depression

Environmental overload

    Loud, busy places

    Too much clutter, lack of routine

    Anything that requires too much thinking, organizing, remembering

New places or people

    Situations that hold no cues to anything familiar

    Situations that trigger fear of failure, embarrassment, or being lost

Complicated demands/jobs that set them up to fail

Activities that require lost skills in planning, starting, organizing, and completing

Activities that involve too many steps

Activities that require new learning

Social situations

Frustration at being unable to say what he or she means

Frustration at being unable to understand caregiver's directions

Feelings of being put down or nervousness

SUPPORTING FAMILIES IN MEETING RESIDENTS' SEXUALITY AND INTIMACY NEEDS

"Emotional security, self-esteem, trust and physical closeness are all important elements in how we feel about ourselves and how we behave with others. Attending to these needs is an important part of caring about and for the person with Alzheimer's disease" (Ballard & Poer, 1993, p. 11). The nursing facility staff can support the family and increase the family's capacity and comfort level in addressing these needs. The following recommendations provide a framework for staff:

- Legitimize sexuality and the importance of intimacy for the caregiver as well as the resident. When sexual needs are normalized, families are able to cope with difficult and unfamiliar behaviors in the resident.
- Help families understand that neither the resident nor they are to blame for sexual behaviors that are inappropriate or unacceptable in the nursing facility setting.
- Empower families to "let go." Spouses may need help in resolving old promises such as "I will never put you in a nursing home." Guilt, grief, anger, and fear become barriers to intimacy and affection. Teaching families to identify their strengths (e.g., sustained care, affection, concern), how to listen, and how to nurture empowers them to give emotionally to the resident. Much of this seems obvious, but simplicity belies the importance of these skills, which become difficult under the stresses of caregiving. For example, communication that is basic to most relationships becomes increasingly difficult for the resident. Teaching families to interpret and use nonverbal communication and to be comfortable with sitting in silence help to create an atmosphere for intimacy.
- Involve families in short-term goals for their relative with dementia. Some families may wish to sit in on care planning conferences. Provide them with specific instructions in how they can help to personalize caregiving. Family members can give back rubs and help with shampooing, shaving, massaging, and rubbing powder or lotion on the skin. These "feel-good" experiences not

only offer physical health benefits but do wonders for the resident's emotional needs as well.

- Share with families the facility's care philosophy for people with dementia; families place a high value on staff who have dementia-specific skills but also who are kind, caring, patient, and understanding with them and their loved one.
- Help the family widen the circle of affection. Encourage and suggest specific roles for children, extended family members, and friends as a conscious attempt to meet the intimacy needs of the resident.
- Help caregivers cope with the painful realities of loss. As the resident becomes increasingly demented, some families may need help in understanding how the disease affects the individual and how to respond to the changes they see.
- Provide the caregiver spouse, in particular, with an opportunity to vent difficult feelings when there has been a limited opportunity to do so. For example: "Friends and family say I am lucky. I still have him with me. He hasn't recognized me in 6 years!" "I am married and yet I am not married. It's hell being in this limbo." "Some of my friends say I should start dating again. I haven't dated since we were both 18. I wouldn't know what to do."

VISITS: AN OFTEN-NEGLECTED OPPORTUNITY FOR PLANNED INTIMACY

Visits are an ideal time and vehicle for creating an atmosphere of intimacy and affection and are a chance to renew and maintain ties to others outside the nursing facility. Visits should provide an opportunity for intimate sexual activity for the resident and his or her spouse/life partner where there is interest and there are no counterindications. Couples have the right to privacy and the freedom to use that time and space as they like. Some individuals report appreciating a private space simply to talk or to be left alone.

Visits are also an opportunity for nonsexual physical intimacy—intimate personal care tasks such as brushing the resident's hair, rubbing his or her back, putting lotion or oils on the skin, hugging spontaneously, dancing, walking, and spending time with the family pet (if allowed) and/or with small children. Many visitors, however, are at a loss as to what to do or what to say. Neither the resident's nor the family's needs are met under such awkward and anxious circumstances. A visiting spouse or adult child, for example, may insist on forcing logic or historical truth when the resident is no longer capable of remembering with clarity, and this creates unnecessary stress in the interaction. When the behavioral symptom of the resident is, for example, confabulation (i.e., making up stories), the response of the family may be impatience and wasted effort in trying to make the person "remember." A daughter reports, "I wish someone had told me to just accept my mom as she was. I would visit her in the nursing home and spend my time trying to correct her confused version of things that weren't even important.

This only frustrated me and made her mad." Other families are more tolerant of the resident's skewed views. They are flexible and creative in adapting to the limitations of the person with dementia, creating a supportive milieu, which, in turn, allows the individual to develop his or her own way of coping. This freedom is essential: Perceived mastery and control of one's environment are important to maintaining self-esteem, even in people with cognitive impairment. A granddaughter shares, "We soon realized that my grandmother readily accepted being in the nursing home and having people attend to her needs because she thought she was in a Palm Beach hotel." Family members supported her enjoyment and acceptance of her new surroundings by assuring her that these "amenities" were paid for and that she should continue to enjoy them.

Good care of residents with dementia promotes the concept of their continued worth as individuals regardless of impairment. Caring staff have available to them many ways to build self-esteem and recognize the special characteristics and accomplishments of people while being careful not to emphasize their present deficits or reduced capacity. Display cases (memory box; see Chapter 8, Figure 4) featuring mementos, pictures, brief bibliographic materials about the life and accomplishments of the people featured, bulletin boards featuring current information about residents (e.g., birthdays, anniversaries, birth of a new grandchild), and residents' arts and crafts are all ways to enhance feelings of worth, to show appreciation for their unique personhood, and to say to residents, *you are special* (Ballard & Gwyther, 1990).

CONCLUSION

Sexuality, intimacy, and the opportunity to form meaningful relationships with others are important needs for all adults, even those who are ill, old, or dependent. The challenge for professional and family caregivers is to maintain the highest quality of life and well-being for those individuals who have a right and who express an interest in affection and intimate relationships, including sexual intimacy, but whose cognitive impairments may preclude appropriate and acceptable ways to get these needs met.

Nursing facilities and families have complementary roles in maintaining the emotional well-being of residents with dementia: Each in different ways can help to buffer residents' feelings of isolation, loneliness, fear, abandonment, and of being unwanted. Staff benefit from education regarding the uniquely individual factors in the sexual behaviors, needs, and interests of people, and from training in responding to those needs in an appropriate, helpful manner. Often uncertain of their roles, families—particularly spouses/life partners—benefit from support, instruction, and validation in ways that they can continue intimacy and meaningful relationships in the nursing facility, however those are defined for the people involved.

REFERENCES

Alzheimer's Association. (1992). *Guidelines for dignity: Goals of specialized Alzheimer/dementia care in residential settings.* Chicago: Author.

Ballard, E.L. (1996). Sexuality in the special care unit. In S.B. Hoffman & M. Kaplan (Eds.), *Special care programs for people with dementia* (pp. 79–99). Baltimore: Health Professions Press.

Ballard, E.L., & Gwyther, L.P. (1990). *Optimum care of the nursing home resident with Alzheimer's disease: "Giving a little extra."* Durham, NC: Joseph and Kathleen Bryan Alzheimer's Disease Research Center, Duke University Center for the Study of Aging.

Ballard, E.L., & Poer, C.M. (1993). *Sexuality and the Alzheimer's patient.* Durham, NC: Joseph and Kathleen Bryan Alzheimer's Disease Research Center, Duke University Center for the Study of Aging.

Bell, V., & Troxel, D. (1997). *The best friends approach to Alzheimer's care.* Baltimore: Health Professions Press.

Burger, S.G., Fraser, V., Hunt, S., & Frank, B. (1996). *Nursing homes: Getting good care there. A consumer action manual prepared by the National Citizens' Coalition for Nursing Home Reform.* San Luis Obispo, CA: Impact Publishers.

George, L.K., & Weiler, S.J. (1981). Sexuality in middle and late life. *Archives of General Psychiatry, 38,* 919–923.

Gwyther, L.P. (1997). *"Home is where I remember things": A curriculum for home and community care.* Durham, NC: Duke University Medical Center, with North Carolina Department of Human Resources, Division of Aging.

Hoffman, S.B., Platt, C.A., & Barry, K.E. (1987, July/August). Managing the difficult dementia patient: The impact on untrained nursing home staff. *American Journal of Alzheimer's Care and Related Disorders & Research, 4*(2), 26–31.

Kaplan, H.S. (1991). Sex therapy with older patients. In W.A. Myers (Ed.), *New techniques in the psychotherapy of older patients* (pp. 21–37). Washington, DC: American Psychiatric Press.

Kuhn, D.R., Greiner, D., & Arsenault, L. (in press). Addressing hypersexuality in Alzheimer's disease. *Journal of Gerontological Nursing.*

Mace, N.L. (1987, Spring). Principles of activities for persons with dementia. *Physical and Occupational Therapy in Geriatrics, 5*(3), 13–27.

Malatesta, V.J. (1989). Sexuality and the older adult: An overview with guidelines for the health care professional. *Journal of Women & Aging, 1*(4), 93–118.

Smith, D.B. (1995, May/June). Staffing and managing special care units for Alzheimer's patients. *Geriatric Nursing, 16*(3), 124–127.

Starkman, E.M. (1993). *Learning to sit in the silence. A journal of caretaking.* Watsonville, CA: Papier-Mache Press.

Starr, B.D. (1985). Sexuality and aging. *Annual Review of Gerontology and Geriatrics, 5,* 97–126.

APPENDIX

SEXUAL BEHAVIOR PROBLEMS AND CONCERNS IN THE NURSING FACILITY: NORTH CAROLINA NURSING FACILITY OMBUDSMEN SURVEY

This questionnaire is intended to be a guide for your responses. Please feel free to expand on the areas listed below or to add an area that you deem important. You do not need to sign your name.

1. This is an area that needs more attention. ____ Yes ____ No

2. How many situations regarding problems of a sexual nature have you encountered during the course of your career? _____

3. Who brought the problem to your attention? ____ Resident ____ Staff ____ Family ____ Other (explain circumstances) _____

4. Did you feel competent to handle the situation? ____ Yes ____ No

5. Have you had training in this area? ____ Yes ____ No

6. Do you agree that special training in sexuality is necessary to respond to problematic sexual behaviors in the nursing facility? ____ Yes ____ No

7. Briefly describe a challenging sexual concern you have confronted in a nursing facility. _____

8. How was the problem resolved? _____

9. From your perspective, what is(are) the most frequently reported problem(s)? _____

10. Typically, how are these problems resolved in the nursing facility? _____ _____

11. Do you agree with how sexual problems are handled in the nursing facility? ____ Yes ____ No

    If not, how would you change this aspect of nursing facility life? _____ _____

12. What topics would you expect to see included in a manual or training materials on sexual concerns in nursing facilities? _____

13. What are the ethical, moral, religious, legal, and cultural concerns of greatest relevance to you? _____

Index

Page numbers followed by "f" indicate figures; page numbers followed by "t" indicate tables.

Families—*continued*
  as caregivers
    changing role of, 89–90, 252
    in late-stage dementia, 212–213
    control issues, 96, 101–102
    and enhanced nurturing, 69
    and FIC protocols, *see* Family
      Involvement in Care
    life before institutional placement, 92
    and partnership with staff, 50
      appropriate responses, 95
      and behavior management plan,
        233–234
      defusing negative emotions, 96–97
      following-through, 97
      importance of, 90
      problem solving, 95–97
      stress-relieving, 91
      supporting, 250–251
      therapeutic environment, creating,
        241
      see also FIC protocols
    stresses on, 91–93, 99–100
      assessment, 94–95
      staff consideration of, 102
    visits, 251–252
Family Involvement in Care (FIC) proto-
    cols, 90, 97–101
  benefits of, 98
  Family and Staff Statement of
    Partnership Intent, 99
  Family–Staff Partnership Contract, for-
    mal, 99, 100–101
    evaluation, periodic, 100–101
    renegotiation of, 101
  education of family members, 99–100
  goals, 98
  orientation to facility, 98
  partnering with staff, 98–99
Fatigue, 144t, 236
Fecal impaction, and agitation, 128–129,
    156
Feeding
  assistive devices, use of in, 202t–203t,
    211t
  finger foods as alternative to, 224
  capabilities of residents

empowering residents' abilities,
    193–196, 205t
  empowering staff, 195–196
CAT order, 205t
cognitive challenges/interventions in,
    196–197
  communication deficits, 201t
  forgetfulness/disorientation,
    198t–199t
  judgment/safety, 199t–200t
  limited attention span, 199t
  perceptual dysfunction, 200t–201t
consistency in, 201t
environmental challenges/interventions
    in, 197
  dining area/equipment, 211t
  overstimulation, 210t
  understimulation, 210t
finger foods, 198, 203t, 224–225
flexibility in, 194
LifeStory Book, 194, 201t, 214–216
and nurturing caregivers, 65
physical challenges/interventions in,
    197
  eating mechanics, 203t–204t
  excess disabilities, 202t–203t
  unproductive movement/noise, 204t
  weight gain/loss, 204t–205t
premorbid preferences, 194, 201t
psychosocial/emotional challenges/inter-
    ventions, 197
  anxiety, 206t–207t
  apathy, 207t
  depression, 207t
  family relationships, 208t–209t
  fearfulness, 206t
  mind-set, problematic, 209t–210t
  pride, 207t–208t
recipes, 225–226
successful, 194, 195–196
techniques, 195–196
  facilitation techniques, 196, 200t, 203t
  tube feeding, 212
  see also Self-feeding
Feeding Behavior Inventory, 162t
FIC, *see* Family Involvement in Care
    protocols

Related Titles Available from Health Professions Press

Special Care Programs for People with Dementia, edited by Stephanie B. Hoffman, Ph.D., & Mary Kaplan, M.S.W.   No. 0335 / $28.95

Interventions for Alzheimer's Disease: A Caregiver's Complete Reference, by Ruth M. Tappen, Ph.D., R.N.   No. 2394 / $35.00

Caring for People with Alzheimer's Disease: A Training Manual for Direct Care Providers, by Gayle Andresen, R.N.-C, M.S., A.N.P./G.N.P.   No. 022X / $26.95

The Best Friends Approach to Alzheimer's Care, by Virginia Bell, M.S.W., & David Troxel, M.P.H.   No. 0351 / $24.95

The Validation Breakthrough: Simple Techniques for Communicating with People with "Alzheimer's-Type Dementia," by Naomi Feil, M.S.W.   No. 0114 / $22.95

Abuse, Neglect, and Exploitation of Older Persons: Strategies for Assessment and Intervention, edited by Lorin Baumhover, Ph.D., and S. Colleen Beall, Dr.P.H.
                    No. 0297 / $29.00

Prices are subject to change.

Please Send Me the Following Books:

Stk No.	Author	Title	Qty	Price
				TOTAL

❏ Check or money order (payable to Health Professions Press)
❏ Bill my institution (attach purchase order)
❏ MasterCard   ❏ VISA   ❏ American Express

Card No. _____   Exp. date_____/_____

Signature _____

Name _____

Address _____

City/State/ZIP _____   Day Phone (____)_____

❏ Please send me a copy of your current catalog.

Health Professions Press   P.O Box 10624   Baltimore, MD   21285-0624
Toll Free (888) 337-8808   Fax (410) 337-8539
E-mail   hpp@pbrookes.com   2KP